W9-ATT-554

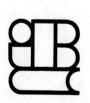

Transforming
Healthcare Organizations

Ellen Marszalek-Gaucher
Richard J. Coffey

Transforming Healthcare Organizations

How to Achieve and Sustain Organizational Excellence

Jossey-Bass Publishers · San Francisco

TRANSFORMING HEALTHCARE ORGANIZATIONS
How to Achieve and Sustain Organizational Excellence
by Ellen Marszalek-Gaucher and Richard J. Coffey

Copyright © 1990 by: Jossey-Bass Inc., Publishers
350 Sansome Street
San Francisco, California 94104

Library of Congress Cataloging-in-Publication Data

Marszalek-Gaucher, Ellen, date.
    Transforming healthcare organizations : how to achieve and sustain organizational excellence / Ellen Marszalek-Gaucher, Richard J. Coffey. — 1st ed.
       p. cm. — (The Jossey-Bass health series)
    Includes bibliographical references.
    Includes index.
    ISBN 1-55542-250-0 (alk. paper)
    1. Health facilities — Administration.   2. Medical care — Quality control.   I. Coffey, Richard James, date.   II. Title.
III. Series.
    [DNLM: 1. Delivery of Health Care — organization & administration — United States.   2. Health Facilities — organization & administration — United States.   3. Health Services — organization & administration — United States.   4. Quality Assurance, Health Care — United States.   WX 27 AA1 M3t]
RA971.M359   1990
362.1'1'068 — dc20
DNLM/DLC
for Library of Congress   90-4777
                                           CIP

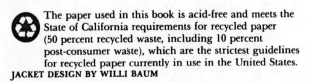

JACKET DESIGN BY WILLI BAUM

FIRST EDITION
HB Printing   10 9 8 7 6 5

*The Jossey-Bass
Health Series*

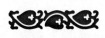

Contents

Preface

Healthcare issues are at the forefront of public debate in the United States. The increasing use of technology and escalating costs of healthcare services have led to debates about their costs versus their benefits. Several initiatives by federal and state governments, insurance companies and other third-party payers, and business corporations are aimed at controlling costs while improving or maintaining services at acceptable levels. Despite providers' and third-party payers' attempts to reduce costs during the last several years, healthcare services continue to be viewed as unnecessarily expensive.

The whole healthcare environment is in a state of flux, and healthcare organizations are under extreme pressure to change. The mode of operation for many organizations is survival. Competition is a reality, and services are being offered in new, less-costly settings, such as ambulatory clinics, work sites, and homes. Diversification and integration strategies are eliminating historical separations of activities among hospitals, nursing homes, physicians, and other providers.

It is time for bold new strategies and a commitment to excellence. It is time to prove that high-quality healthcare is also cost-efficient care. Organizations that do not change may cause their own demise. The required changes are not a matter of small, incremental reductions in costs. The emphasis must be on eliminating rework, reducing complexity, and understanding variation in quality measurements to reduce cost and add value to services. In order to survive, organizations in the healthcare industry must undergo a major transformation in the ways they relate to their customers and provide services to them. Organizational leaders and managers are the only people who can lead this transformation. But rapid transformation requires new knowledge, attitudes, and leadership skills that today's healthcare executives and managers rarely possess.

Purpose of the Book

We have written *Transforming Healthcare Organizations* to offer specific approaches to making the broad organizational changes called for today within the healthcare industry. This book provides personal guidance and suggests useful ways for leaders, managers, and staff within an organization to develop a vision and a process for continual improvement as well as to learn to communicate effectively with one another and with customers and suppliers. The book conveys our experience of the transformation currently under way at the University of Michigan Hospitals, Ann Arbor, Michigan.

Our aim is to present practical ideas and actions that can begin an organizational transformation. Although the suggested changes in culture and leadership may seem simple, we have found that these changes, integral to transformational success, are very difficult and require several years to implement fully.

Much of the current literature in healthcare and other industries emphasizes bold leadership during times of stress and change. We agree that leadership skills are critical and discuss them at length. However, it is essential to remember that followers are also critical: leaders exist only when there are followers. Therefore, leaders should take action to involve and empower employees so that they will be contributing followers now and good leaders in the future. Employees need leadership, training, tools, and instructions to initiate the necessary grassroots improvements. Leaders should actively involve customers and suppliers to improve the quality and value of the services and products. They should also affirm their commitment to the communities they serve. Most healthcare organizations are unique neighborhood businesses based on a series of doctor-patient relationships.

This book is unique in that it addresses several interdependent components of organizational transformation. It provides specific approaches, actions, and practical examples for each major component of transformation. These strategies can be implemented by managers at different levels of healthcare organizations. The suggested approaches enable managers to initiate proactive leadership in place of the traditional reactive approach.

Audience

The primary audience for *Transforming Healthcare Organizations* is leaders and managers in the healthcare industry. This book is written expressly for them. Included in this group are board members, executives, middle managers, and first-line supervisors. Physicians, nurses, pharmacists, therapists, and other professionals with management responsibilities can also benefit from the information this book provides. Many of the action steps we describe must be implemented by line employees; these are the people who can most directly and immediately transform healthcare organizations in these times of rapidly changing requirements.

The secondary audience is students of healthcare management and healthcare employees aspiring to management roles. These people can benefit from the book because it provides a practical understanding of the issues and functions specific to healthcare organizations. The future of the healthcare industry depends on new practitioners and managers who learn to involve everyone in the pursuit of continual improvement to better meet customer requirements.

Leaders and managers of the following organizations may also find the management principles in this book helpful: health maintenance organizations (HMOs), preferred-provider organizations (PPOs), healthcare suppliers, governmental agencies, insurance companies and third-party payers, professional organizations, review and accreditation organizations, business and industrial organizations, universities, and consulting companies.

Overview of the Contents

In Chapter One, we introduce the challenge of continual improvement and the need for transformation of healthcare organizations. Continual improvement must be integrated into both personal and corporate cultures. In Chapter Two, we describe many changes in the healthcare environment that are serving as catalysts for major changes in expectations, relationships, and reimbursement related to healthcare. Chapter Three specifically describes how to anticipate and adapt to the changing requirements. Chapter Four shows how to revitalize and communicate the mission, vision, and values throughout an organization in terms everyone can understand. Chapter Five presents a step-by-step guide to implementing a total quality process. Quality will be one of the most important and most pursued topics of the 1990s. The public's sensitivity to quality has been raised by advertising and improved products and services in other industries. Healthcare organizations have always been concerned about the quality of clinical care, but this concern must be extended to include all our activities. In this chapter, we discuss specific quality-improvement techniques. Chapter Six addresses actions to promote an organizational culture of continual improvement. It relates W. Edwards Deming's fourteen points for management specifically to the healthcare industry. Chapter Seven focuses on innovation and creativity as a method to improve quality and cost-effectiveness. Transformation is best accomplished by tapping the vast knowledge of all the people working in our organizations, not just a few managers at the top. Chapter Eight presents methods for reorganizing the way work is accomplished. These new work methods will require major changes in the way we organize, work together, and relate to work associates. We must pursue and develop a multicultural work force more broadly representative of the racial and ethnic groups of the population served—one in which people directly performing jobs have greater input than before into process improvements. Chapter Nine compares organizational success to individual definitions of success, and identifies typical barriers to success. It offers actions for everyone that promotes both individual and organizational success. Chapter Ten presents twenty action steps to improve the cost-effectiveness of a department or organization. Chapter Eleven points out the need for better information to manage more effectively as the acuity of inpatients increases, lengths of stay decrease, services are geographically diversified, and reimbursement is restricted. Such an environment requires rapid management responses. The chapter presents better ways to use quantitative and qualitative information in decision making. Chapter Twelve provides strategies and actions for improving leadership effectiveness. It describes the specific knowledge, attitudes, and skills leaders need, along with specific actions that can be taken to develop those attributes necessary to lead the transformation. Chapter Thirteen concludes with a summary of several approaches that will ensure continuing organizational success. A resource section at the end of the book extracts the action steps discussed in the chapters.

Acknowledgments

Many people contributed to the creation of this book, and we wish to thank them. John D. Forsyth, chief executive officer of the University of Michigan Hospitals, is a visionary leader who taught us to listen intently to our employees and involve them in planning for the future. He set the tone for our philosophy of transformation. During preparation of the manuscript, we were assisted in our research and editing by Richard E. Finger, John Gialanella, Neal E. Gilbert, Lisa L. Hodgson, Anthony E. Keck, James M. Molloy, and Laura E. User. Anthony, James, Laura, and Lisa helped us with much-needed research support. We also wish to thank the friends and colleagues who reviewed drafts of the manuscript and helped us to shape it: Karl G. Bartscht, Ann W. Beard, Michael O. Bice, Jeptha Dalston, William Densmore, Mindy Eisenberg, John A. "Jack" Germ, Lillian Goodman, Rebecca L. McGovern, Lynn O'Neal, Kenneth G. Peltzie, Richard Redman, Linda Rodgers, and Patricia A. Warner. They provided valuable ideas to improve the book.

Finally, we thank our families, who were understanding of

our need to write this book. We appreciate their support. Our children also demonstrated great patience during the process, for which we are thankful. We hope that in some small way this book will serve as an inspiration for them to pursue their creative interests. We would like to dedicate this book to our families: Oneta, Todd, and Tonya Coffey and Steve Gaucher and the Marszalek/Gaucher children.

Ann Arbor, Michigan   Ellen Marszalek-Gaucher
June 1990   Richard J. Coffey

The Authors

Ellen Marszalek-Gaucher is senior associate hospital director and chief operating officer of the University of Michigan Hospitals in Ann Arbor, Michigan, a large academic health center with several satellite facilities and over $500 million in annual revenues. She also has a faculty appointment in the University of Michigan School of Nursing. Marszalek-Gaucher is a registered nurse who received her B.S. degree (1975) from Worcester State College in nursing and her M.S.P.H. degree (1977) from Clark University. She has completed other postgraduate education at Boston University and the University of Michigan.

Her most recent research has been in the area of enhancing organizational innovation and creativity and in leading a total quality management process for the University of Michigan Hospitals. Marszalek-Gaucher serves on the advisory board of the National Demonstration Project on Quality Improvement in Health Care funded by the John A. Hartford Foundation and the Harvard Community Health Plan. She is also on the editorial board of *Health Care Competition Week*.

Marszalek-Gaucher has fifteen years of experience in senior management positions in healthcare organizations. Her previous positions were director of nursing and associate hospital director of ambulatory care at the University of Michigan and assistant director of nursing and director of ambulatory care at the University of Massachusetts. She has published numerous articles, served as a consultant, and lectured nationally in the field of hospital management and systems development.

Richard J. Coffey is director of management systems at the University of Michigan Hospitals, Ann Arbor; lecturer in industrial and operations engineering at the University of Michigan; and president of Coffey Associates in Milan, Michigan. He received his B.S.E. degree (1967) from the University of Michigan in industrial engineering and his M.S. degree (1971) from the University of Arizona in systems engineering. He holds an M.S.E. degree (1972) and a Ph.D. degree (1975), both from the University of Michigan in industrial and operations engineering.

Coffey's current activities include development, training, and project support for a total quality process and decision support services for senior managers within the University of Michigan Medical Center. He has performed operations analysis and planning and market research projects in a number of university, consulting, government, insurance, and private organizations within the healthcare industry since 1963 and has worked in foreign countries as well as in the United States. He received an industrial engineering Alpha Pi Mu honor membership in 1966, a special research fellowship from the National Center for Health Services Research and Development from 1971 to 1974, and a first-place literature award from the Hospital Management Systems Society in 1979 (with K. G. Bartscht) for "Management Engineering—A Method to Improve Productivity," an article in *Topics in Health Care Financing*. Dr. Coffey has authored over twenty published articles and a chapter in the book *Health Care Delivery Planning* (1973). He has given many presentations at regional and national conferences in addition to his extensive project presentations.

Transforming
Healthcare Organizations

Chapter One

The Challenge of Organizational Excellence in Healthcare Organizations

This book is for all those who seek to understand and manage change, as a way of building a better future. In these competitive times, healthcare managers must establish an organizational culture of continual improvement to enhance their ability to compete. This means constantly challenging every system, process, service, and product so that quality is built in from the beginning. Planning for quality reduces costs and avoids quality-by-inspection, a much more expensive option.

To develop a focus on quality will require change in the culture of most healthcare organizations. We in healthcare pride ourselves on being experts in quality assurance, but we have too often been satisfied to treat the symptoms of poor quality instead of treating the underlying disease.

Changing an organizational culture is difficult because the task involves behavior patterns, beliefs, and all the other aspects of work and thought that are characteristic of people in groups, including organizations. Executives and managers have often tried to implement sweeping changes without regard for the values and norms of their organizations. Such changes have fallen far short of their original goals.

Changing the culture is particularly difficult in a healthcare organization because professional interests and departmental subcultures often conflict with institutional goals. The best way to facilitate lasting change is to spend time imagining the ideal new culture — discussing the barriers that may preclude its development and planning how to get from where you are to where you should be.

To shape the new culture, you must first understand the

existing one. It is important to evaluate your environment and determine any beliefs and values that employees share. You must also spend time reviewing the values that will help you create the kind of healthcare organization you desire. You must move the organization away from its focus on how things are done now and toward a more ideal state. Leaders must develop and present a vision for the future that is compelling enough for people to endure the changes that will be required. The leaders need to guide people by fully describing the vision and the plans for change and by involving them in the change process (for example, through focus groups, open workshops, and employee meetings).

Discussions and focus groups can help in building consensus on the general direction and values that will guide the organization. Once the new direction is set, leaders should recognize and reward values and behaviors that move the organization closer to its ideal. This policy will enhance the quality of care in the organization and allow the transformation to begin.

In our experience, management is responsible for the success or failure of an organization. Management therefore has primary responsibility for transforming any organization. We hope to provide ideas that will improve the management of your healthcare organization and get you started on the road to continual improvement. Throughout the book, specific Action Steps are highlighted to help you begin building a culture of continual improvement. A summary of the Action Steps appears in the Resource. We have used the Action Steps successfully and observed them in use. They work.

Change: The Only Constant

Why build a culture of continual improvement? Our environment demands it; our industry is in evolution. There have been more changes in the 1980s than during any other time in the history of healthcare. In fact, change seems to be the only constant in today's challenging environment. After almost two decades of growth, low financial risk, and autonomy, healthcare executives are facing new ground rules and different incentives. Operating margins from inpatient services have declined by millions of dollars, turning highly profitable organizations into marginal ones and marginal organizations into failures. This financial crisis has caused grave concern among healthcare executives and trustees. A survey of healthcare executives (Touche Ross & Company, 1988) reported widespread pessimism about the future; half of the 1,419 executives polled said that their institutions risked failure in the next five years.

The turmoil in the industry has led to increasing turnover of healthcare executives. According to Bell (1988, p. 19), "The AHA [American Hospital Association], American College of Healthcare Executives and the executive search firm of Heidrick and Struggles found that 24.2% of hospital CEOs left their positions from 1986 to 1987, compared to 16.9% from 1981 to 1982." By the end of 1988, administrative turnover had reached an annual rate of 25 to 30 percent, leaving trustees and new management teams struggling to keep their institutions on an even keel. When things take a turn for the worse, there is a better approach than having boards change leaders or executives change jobs; it is to understand why the organization is not competing well and what needs to change.

In the hospital industry, we cannot have business as usual. Fundamental change is necessary—a complete transformation, if you will—for organizations to compete effectively in an increasingly demanding marketplace.

Competition and Revenue Reduction

Everyone in our industry would agree that the business of running a healthcare organization has become more complex. Some, however, are content to blame the federal government, other payers, or the advent of prospective payment systems for their problems. This is a mistake. One must look at all the changes and their impacts on the organization and then develop an overall strategy, with substrategies for specific changes.

Competition among providers has been responsible for the erosion of business. Competition is coming from old

Table 1. Competition Among Healthcare Providers.

Type of Provider	Examples
Hospital	Single hospital
	Multihospital group
Physician	Individual physician
	Group practice
Alternative financing system	Health maintenance organization
	Preferred-provider organization
	Blue Cross/Blue Shield trust
	Medical care foundation
	Insurance company
Specialty provider	Ambulatory-care center
	Freestanding location
	Location in shopping center
	Ambulatory-surgery center
	Cancer center
	Comprehensive rehabilitation center
	Diet center
	Eyecare center
	Franchised medical/health center
	Dialysis center
	Psychiatric center
	Home care
	High-tech care (e.g., infusion therapy)
	Home-care agency
	Imaging center
	Physical therapy practice
	Plastic surgery center
	Psychiatric program
	Urgent-care center
	Visiting nurse agency
	Women's center

sources, as well as from a variety of new market entrants, as shown in Table 1. For example, hospitals find that their traditional "bread and butter" revenue-producing services (such as radiology, pathology, pharmaceutical supplies, and ambulatory surgery) are being offered by many other healthcare providers at competitive prices (see Table 2). Increased competition within and among healthcare segments has created a marketplace foreign to many longtime providers.

To plot strategy for the future, a competitive analysis is

Table 2. Threatened Sources of Hospital Revenue.

Major Sources of Revenue and Profit	Threats
Acute inpatient care	Dramatic changes in level of demand, coverage, methods of payment, methods of service delivery
	Rationing based on financial limitations, physicians' restriction of care
Routine surgical procedures	Competition from new market entrants (ambulatory-surgical centers, physicians' group practices, urgent-care centers)
	Required second opinions to reduce surgery
Ancillary services	Competition from specialists (orthopedic surgeons offering physical therapy, radiologists with imaging centers), contract management companies, physicians' offices, new market entrants

critical. You must know with whom your organization is competing for which services and products, and you must measure your quality and price against the competition's. An analysis will help you target your portfolio of services and products. Unless there are more important social or educational considerations, your goal should be learning to compete and to replace unprofitable services and products with those that can offer a positive margin.

Crisis or Opportunity for Leaders

Healthcare leaders are scrambling for ways to operate in an increasingly chaotic and ambiguous environment. Toffler's (1970) message — that change causes anxiety — is as relevant today as when *Future Shock* was published. According to Bennis and Nanus (1985, p. 13), "The contexts of apathy, escalating change and uncertainty make leadership like maneuvering over ever faster and more undirected ball bearings." Providing organizational leadership during times of revolutionary change can be extremely stressful. As the healthcare industry becomes more competitive, there will be many new problems.

Because the environmental changes are so intense, it is important to maintain a broad view of the healthcare industry. The pressure to decrease length of stay in hospitals offers many opportunities for subacute-care providers (such as skilled- and custodial-care nursing homes, home-care agencies, and visiting nurse agencies) to expand their services. Many services are now being reimbursed only if they are provided on an outpatient basis, and this arrangement offers opportunities for expansion of ambulatory-care centers and physicians' group practices. If one remains alert to the broad range of possible services in a variety of settings, each crisis may become an opportunity.

Changes in planning represent a huge transformation. In the past, planning meant keeping up with the Joneses. For example, when your competition opened a sports medicine service, you opened one, too. Planning must now include diversification, downsizing, and elimination of unprofitable services. For Tichy and Devanna (1986a, p. 4), "beating the competition is exhilarating, but it's painful to lay off workers, sell off businesses and disrupt traditions." This environment brings many ethical dilemmas as managers try to compete.

When old strategies and tactics do not work, one way of dealing with the ambiguity is to find an example or a model with which to build a new frame of reference. We believe that one such model can be found in the transformations that are occurring in many American companies. These transformations have been brought about by leaders who saw the need for reinvention and began systematically to renew and revitalize their organizations so that they could respond to their markets more appropriately and less expensively. These leaders sought out change. They recognized that specific events in an environment make it possible to bring about a major reorganization that can focus on making good things better. This insight contrasts with the attitude that seems to exist during stable times: "If it ain't broke, don't fix it."

Challenging times allow leaders to come forward and set a new direction, with excellence as a goal. According to

Hickman and Silva (1984, p. 23), "Individuals who have developed specific skills create superior organizational performance. Excellence doesn't happen miraculously but springs from pacesetting levels of personal effectiveness and efficiency." If you desire organizational transformation, you must recognize the need for changes, develop a bold plan, actively sponsor the changes, and support them tenaciously over periods of time.

The Need for Transformation in Healthcare

In the early 1980s, some management authors began to call for a new type of leadership, to enhance America's ability to compete in world markets. These authors interviewed leaders who have made a dramatic difference in their companies (Tichy and Devanna, 1986a, 1986b; Peters and Waterman, 1982; Hickman and Silva, 1984; Naisbitt and Aburdene, 1985). Business leaders tell us that during times of decline, the speed and impact of change have often been underestimated. Time to plan was considered a luxury, and only companies with a bias for action were able to assume positions of industry leadership. Therefore, they developed a new style of leadership, facilitated the development of new products, and, through innovation, invaded new markets. They stressed customer satisfaction (to establish loyalty), and they pruned the work force to enhance productivity and cost-effectiveness. Quality not only became the new golden word, it became a new way of life.

Successful leaders in industry, responding to the global economy, have begun to renew and revitalize their organizations, and healthcare leaders must do the same. Hospital leaders, in particular, must begin by retreating from shrinking markets, dropping unneeded and unprofitable programs and services, and leading their organizations toward new products and services, diversification, and process improvements that will raise quality and lower costs.

Most important, leaders must keep their eyes on the customers, both external and internal. They must work with their communities to decide which services will be added, deleted, and modified. At the same time, they must restructure work and reduce the work force. They must motivate their employees to help in achieving this reinvention through participatory and intelligently planned change.

From current research, we know that innovations do not necessarily come from leaders. They also come from customers, workers, and researchers. The transforming leader knows how to listen to others, actively foster employees' participation, and solicit many alternative solutions (Kouzes and Posner, 1987). Transforming leaders continually seek data and ideas, to avoid being locked into old ways of doing things. They have learned how to tap the creative potential of employees and customers. They ask the right questions and try to visualize each problem from a variety of perspectives. Transforming leaders integrate information with the advantages and disadvantages of different alternatives, to choose the best ones overall.

These types of leaders have been given many names. Kanter (1983) calls them "change masters." Kaiser (1981a) calls them "future makers." Burns (1978) calls them "transformational leaders." Conger, Kanungo, and Associates (1988) call them "charismatic leaders." The name is less important than the concept of extraordinary leadership.

The cover story of the *Hospitals* magazine published May 20, 1987, asked, "What Is Leadership? What Is Impeding It?" (Sabatino, 1987). Just fifteen years ago, the health field had few chief executive officers (CEOs); its leaders were administrators. Although the field has always been open to change, evolution was more the norm, and few associated the words *bold* and *decisive* with healthcare leaders. In this new age, when survival is key, it is clear that healthcare leaders must be bold and decisive, both at the midmanagement level and at the top of the organization.

One note of caution — you cannot achieve transformation by yourself. No matter what your position within a healthcare organization, the steps are the same. You must develop a vision for the future, create an environment for change, and convince others to join you in making the vision a reality. You must actively educate everyone involved with your organization, especially the board of directors, to recognize the rapid changes and help develop appropriate responses to change.

> *Action Step*: **Become more proactive by providing regular education to the board of directors, executives, physicians, managers, employees, suppliers, and customers about the changing environment and the actions required to make improvements.**

Definitions of Successful Organizations

One of the biggest challenges during times of rapid change is changing our measures of success.

Historical Success Measures

Historically, the indicators of success for a healthcare organization have included the factors discussed in the sections that follow.

Acute Inpatient-Care Focus. The liberal payment for acute inpatient care, and lower per-case income for ambulatory care, have led most organizations to focus on the acute inpatient-care side of the business. In fact, the term *hospital* was once synonymous with organized medical care; there was little attention paid to services for healthy individuals.

Number of Beds. In the past, the number of a hospital's or long-term-care facility's beds was viewed as an indication of its success. It was common to judge an administrator of a five-hundred-bed hospital as more successful than an administrator of a three-hundred-bed hospital, even if only three hundred of the five hundred beds were being used. This tendency, plus the difficulty of relicensing beds, has led many institutions to continue operating more licensed beds than required.

Number of Patient Days. Since many third-party payers reimbursed on a per-diem basis or on the basis of incurred costs, institutions with more patient days were generally more successful, even if the average length of stay was longer than required or longer than the national or regional average.

Gross Revenues. In the past, institutions with larger gross revenues were judged to be more successful than those with smaller gross revenues. With third-party payers implementing fixed-price payments and large discounts, however, gross revenue is no longer a good measure of success.

The "More Is Better" Axiom. In the past, more of anything was generally viewed as "better." Examples were everywhere: more inpatient days, more lab tests, more X-ray exams, more surgery. Since we billed for each exam and procedure and judged our success according to our revenue, physicians who ordered the most tests were considered to be the most valuable to the institution. Similarly, department managers who increased the volume of services were viewed as more successful, even if the services were unnecessary.

Number of Staff Managed. A manager who increased the number of staff working in his or her department was generally rewarded with a salary increase to reflect the increased "responsibility." Likewise, many human resource departments have used the number of staff being supervised as an important criterion for determining job grade and salary. Thus, the incentive was to increase staff, since success was judged according to the number of staff managed.

Low-Risk Stability. In most healthcare organizations, managers have earned success by avoiding risks and maintaining the status quo. A person championing change was often viewed as a problem employee who did not fit the mold.

To move from being an organization whose motto is "More is better" to being a streamlined, competitive organization is a major transition. Because change has been so rapid and constant during the last five years, many healthcare professionals (such as physicians and nurses) are not fully aware of environmental changes and their impact on organizations. Even if they are aware of changes, however, many professionals need a focus for knowing how to respond and assist the organization.

The leader's role is to educate everyone in the organization about the changing environment and about the need to improve quality, cost-effectiveness, and value. There are difficult trade-offs in the healthcare industry that can be made only by such healthcare professionals as physicians, nurses, and therapists. For example, what is the minimum amount of information required to reach an accurate diagnosis and avoid a malpractice suit? How do we reduce the cost of procedures? Even cursory reviews of healthcare organizations reveal tremendous waste and duplication of services. These issues must be addressed for better use of scarce resources. With the cooperation of the professional healthcare staff, processes can be revamped and waste reduced. Not enough attention has been paid to product evaluation and standardization as an effective method of attaining both quality standardization and cost reduction.

> *Action Step*: **Inform physicians, nurses, and other direct healthcare providers about financial constraints, the need to improve quality and cost-effectiveness, and the need to reduce the cost of procedures and supplies. Involve staff in planning and implementing ideas to improve quality and reduce costs.**

New Measures of Success

When Medicare, Medicaid, and other third-party payers began using diagnosis-related groups (DRGs) and other prospective payment systems during the middle 1980s, financial reimbursement dramatically changed. Payers began reimbursing according to fixed prices for healthcare services, as is common with other kinds of services. Encouraging more exams, tests, procedures, and patient days became a financial disincentive rather than a measure of success.

The measures of success are slowly changing to reflect the new business situation under prospective payment systems. It is still common, however, to hear comparisons of success that are based on the old criteria. Some new and emerging measures of success are described in the following sections, along with some examples.

Profitability and Return on Investment. Healthcare institutions are beginning to look at profitability, financial return on sales, and return on investment as important measures of success. Gross revenue, as traditionally calculated, is of lesser importance. Most hospitals receive from payers only 65 to 75 percent of the amount charged for services, a figure that depends on the mix of payers.

Customers' Loyalty. With increased competition in providing all types of healthcare services and products, customers' and suppliers' loyalty has become an important measure of success. Most hospitals with specialist physicians are concerned about their referral sources, and some are actively expanding their referral networks. This situation has changed how physicians in general practice, family practice, and internal medicine are seen. They are now viewed as important customers, whose loyalty is desired. In the current environment, an organization with strong loyalty from physicians and patients will be judged successful.

Other loyalty-related measures of success involve the referral relationships among providers of different healthcare services and products. Strong collaborative relationships among hospitals, long-term-care facilities, home-care agencies, hospices, equipment suppliers, third-party payers, health maintenance organizations, and other organizations are now considered to indicate success.

Customers' loyalty can be measured by satisfaction surveys. Patient-origin information is another source of information, showing the percentage of patients drawn from selected geographical areas.

Ambulatory Services. A large ambulatory-care volume is viewed as the best way to capture referrals to inpatient facilities, diagnostic services, home-care services, and medical equipment businesses. Organizations with successful ambulatory-care centers do generate inpatient admissions, but the profit margin for ambulatory care is much less than for inpatient care and may increase financial risk if not managed carefully. The axiom "More is better" can also lead to losses in the ambulatory-care setting.

As more costs are shifted to ambulatory-care settings, ambulatory care, like inpatient services, is experiencing increased regulation and competition. For example, some payers reimburse physicians a fixed amount per insured person, per month, for all medical care. If more visits than necessary are scheduled, time and money are lost.

Consumers are seeking convenient services, but most hospitals have not planned ambulatory services with convenience in mind. Hospitals tend to establish ambulatory-care centers to compete with neighboring hospitals, rather than to meet identified needs in the community. Such ventures have been generally less profitable than they were planned to be. Moreover, many hospitals have continued to provide these services at a loss, rather than closing the centers and cutting their losses. In many cases, expansion of ambulatory services has increased hospitals' financial risk, rather than providing new sources of revenue.

The simple act of establishing ambulatory-care centers does not automatically ensure either inpatient referrals or profits. Objectives for these ventures must be very clear, and the centers must be carefully managed. Contrast the following two objectives: If positive contributions were the objective, a center would be established or maintained only if it were profitable; if increasing inpatient referrals were the objective, a loss on the center might be acceptable. In either case, any financial contribution to the hospital that results from referrals should be estimated.

Capable and Committed People. It is trite but true to say that people are our most important asset. Healthcare is a labor-intensive industry; people represent the majority of costs and the greatest opportunity for success in healthcare organizations. In an environment of rapid change, with limited supplies of several types of healthcare professionals, organizations with stable work forces of capable and committed people will be more successful. The number of knowledgeable, experienced people will be a new measure of success in an organization. It is crucial to build a committed work force by involving people in decision making and fostering an institutionwide collaborative spirit.

Clear Vision, Values, and Goals. Although they cannot be quantified, clear vision, values, and goals will be prevalent in successful organizations. These attributes help guide the staff and strengthen commitment to the organization.

Ability to Plan and Change. Success requires an organization to anticipate environmental change and plan strategies to meet the needs of the population while accomplishing its own goals. Given rapidly changing clinical technologies, reimbursement arrangements, and regulations, it is becoming much more important to learn, identify factors and trends, initiate strategies, and adapt to change quickly. Those who can adapt quickly will be more successful.

Facilities. Facilities alone cannot make an organization successful, but they are important in meeting the standards and expectations of our customers. Appropriate facilities are prerequisites of successful competition. Only successful organizations will have the money required to develop and maintain modern facilities.

Characteristics of Successful Organizations

Given the measures of success that we have just discussed, what are the characteristics of successful organizations today? What will they be in the future? We believe that successful organizations can be measured according to the following eleven criteria.

1. *Well-understood mission and values*: As competition and financial constraints become stronger, organizations cannot afford undirected managers or employees. To facilitate achievement of goals, the mission and values that guide the organization should be clear, crisp, and broadly shared.

2. *External focus*: The successful healthcare organization will be sharply focused on its current and potential customers, as well as on its competitors. It will review its community mission frequently and will poll customers often, to be sure that goals stay on track.

3. *Total quality and customer responsiveness*: Successful organizations will be particularly responsive to customers' requirements. For example, NKC Hospitals, Inc., of Louisville, Kentucky, bases departmental and individual goals on the responses received from external and internal customer surveys. Constant measuring of progress toward meeting requirements ensures customer responsiveness.

4. *Capable and committed people:* Successful organizations have well-trained and experienced people who have committed themselves to the organization and its success. It is easier to recruit excellent people to an organization when it already has an excellent staff.

5. *Innovation and creativity*: Successful organizations actively listen to customers' ideas on how to make good services and products even better. By *customers*, we mean employees in the organization, as well as such traditional external customers as patients and physicians. Organizations that regularly listen to customers and seek innovations to be more responsive are on the road to continual improvement.

6. *Market differentiation*: Given the wide variety of customers' requirements, it is impossible for an organization to be all things to all people at all times. Patients and others seek services and products tailored to their own needs, and the success of specialized services and products supports this market-segmentation approach. Examples of specialized services include children's hospitals, women's hospitals and centers, ambulatory surgery centers, kidney dialysis centers, eyecare centers, and rehabilitation centers. The future success of healthcare organizations will depend on their ability to meet specific customers' requirements, rather than pursuing a generalist approach. This type of thinking may also lead to a new definition of healthcare systems, whereby many institutions will collaborate on which ones will offer which services along a continuum, rather than continuing to compete for opportunities to provide a wide range of services.

7. *Empowerment of employees*: Employees are an organization's primary source of knowledge and creativity. In making necessary changes, successful organizations will find ways to involve and empower their employees. For example, reducing the number of levels of management can enhance employees' decision-making authority and willingness to take risks in the search for improved methods of providing patient care or other services or products.

8. *Cost-effectiveness*: Employers, the federal and state governments, third-party payers, patients, and others are all concerned about healthcare costs. Providers — particularly the large-volume, traditional healthcare services — must become more cost-conscious and cost-effective. The best route to improved quality and cost-effectiveness is involvement of everyone in process improvements aimed at eliminating unnecessary work, rework, and waste.

9. *Effective management of information*: Cost-effective management of patient care and of healthcare organizations depends critically on timely, accurate information. For example, it is unnecessarily expensive to keep a patient in the hospital an extra day while waiting for test results or

communication. There is also a need for information to be available at several locations simultaneously. Success will increasingly depend on effective management of clinical and other information.

10. *Adaptability*: The ability to adapt, cope, and manage change consistently will distinguish successful organizations. Such organizations continually review themselves and compare their services and products with the best benchmarks available in the world.

11. *Leadership*: A successful organization will have strong, visionary leadership, with the ability to devise a vision and mobilize the organization to achieve it.

Beckham (1989) identified and reported on characteristics of ten "winning" hospitals. All of the hospitals shared the following characteristics:

- A fortunate confluence of talented physicians, managers and board members
- Meaningful differentiation from competitors
- Consistency, constancy, and concentration of purpose
- Visible leadership
- Purpose and pride
- Advanced clinical capabilities
- Integration of hospitals' and physicians' interests

The ten hospitals are listed below:

Hospital	*CEO/Chairperson(s)*
St. Thomas Hospital, Nashville, Tennessee	Sister Julianna Beuerlein
Beth Israel Hospital, Boston, Massachusetts	Mitch Rabkin, M.D.
Lutheran General Hospital, Park Ridge, Illinois	George Caldwell
HCA Wesley Medical Center, Wichita, Kansas	Jack Davis, Jim Biltz

Tampa General Hospital, Tampa, Florida	Newell France
The Methodist Hospital, Houston, Texas	Larry Mathis
Barnes Hospital, St. Louis, Missouri	Max Poll
Abbott-Northwestern, Minneapolis, Minnesota	Gordon Sprenger
Memorial Medical Center, Long Beach, California	Steven Ummel
Riverside Methodist, Columbus, Ohio	Erie Chapman

Beckham (1989, p. 23) devised the following recommendations after examining these and other successful hospitals in the United States:

> Invest in the very best medical talent. Stamp out monopolies of mediocrity.
> Either be big or be different. Preferably both.
> Leverage bigness into productivity, quality, preference.
> If you're already big, keep others from getting big.
> Keep on track. Avoid fads. Don't be a bunny. Build one success at a time.
> Give your organization a sense of purpose. Lead by example.
> If you're small, crawl in a niche and dig in.
> Give physicians and employees a real sense of ownership.

The challenge seems clear: you must *lead* your organization to compete more effectively.

Chapter Two

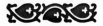

Catalysts for Change in the Healthcare Environment

Several underlying social, economic, and technological changes are affecting our health and the healthcare system. Some of the more important changes are summarized in this chapter, to provide a basis for understanding still other changes and recommendations for dealing with them.

Factors Influencing the Healthcare Environment

Social Expectations

Many changes in social expectations have caused and are causing changes in the healthcare environment.

Perceptions of Social Responsibility. Historically in the United States, there has been a strong sense of families' direct responsibility for their disabled and elderly members. Dual-career families, increased geographical mobility, and decreased size of the extended family have led to a trend of decreasing family responsibility for the healthcare of family members. Today, rather than caring for the person at home, a family may place a disabled child or elderly parent in a nursing home. This tendency increases the need for long-term care and increases the financial burden on Medicare, Medicaid, and other publicly funded programs.

Public Responsibility for Healthcare. In the early 1960s, a change began to take place in the public's perception of healthcare accessibility. In what Starr (1982) has called "the Liberal Years," healthcare came to be viewed as the right of all, rather than the privilege of those who could pay for it. Medicare and Medicaid were enacted in 1965 as federal entitlements for the elderly and the poor. Through new laws, taxpayers became responsible for more of the total U.S. healthcare cost. After these programs were enacted, the healthcare industry grew at a geo-metrical rate.

Healthcare as an Economic Good. With growth in tech-nology, services, and the eligible population, healthcare costs are now unacceptably high. We are seeing yet another shift: healthcare, rather than being viewed as a social good, is now being seen as an economic good. Very few people favor restrict-ing basic and emergency healthcare services, but people in increasing numbers are in favor of limiting optional, expensive, and terminal-care services. Michael Krentz, president of the American College of Emergency Physicians, has stated this so-cioeconomic dilemma succinctly: "On the one hand, we have a moral, ethical and legal obligation to see a patient. Nobody, on the other hand, has a moral or legal obligation to pay for that care" (Ansberry, 1988, pp. 1, A11). The most widely noted changes in public policy to restrict healthcare services are occur-ring in Oregon, which has created a list of medical services and ranked them by importance (Price, 1989). Services ranked as low priorities are not covered by Oregon's Medicaid program.

> *Action Step*: **Become proactively involved in com-munity, state, and professional organizations to seek acceptable solutions to public issues that affect healthcare organizations.**

The Latest Technology. The public has generally become aware of new types of technology through the mass media (television, radio, books, magazines, newspapers) and, more recently, through the advertising of hospitals and clinics. People ask for and expect new technologies to be available in the facilities they use. This demand causes a particular dilemma for small hospitals, long-term-care facilities, and ambulatory-care facilities, which may try to compete by adding costly equipment to satisfy customers, even when volume may be insufficient to produce a satisfactory return on investments at reasonable charges.

These social expectations have changed the way health-care organizations must respond to their customers. In the future, the most successful organizations will be those that adapt to society's and customers' expectations in the most cost-effective manner.

Population and Demographics

Changes in population and demographics both result from and affect the healthcare system. Life expectancy has increased steadily, and that increase is projected to continue. One of every nine Americans is over age sixty-five; by the year 2010, the proportion will be one in five (Coile, 1986b; Schick, 1986). Elderly people have the highest rates of hospitalization and the longest lengths of stay. The demand for ambulatory care, acute inpatient care, and long-term care will expand dramatically, given increased use of healthcare services among the elderly.

Improved Quality of Life and Extended Life Expectancy. Modern medicine has improved the quality of life for many people. Ear surgery can help hearing-impaired persons to hear better. A coronary bypass graft can allow someone with debilitating heart disease and pain to return to work. Joint replacement lets people continue to be mobile and to work, rather than remaining disabled for the rest of their lives. Neonatal care has increased the survival rate of premature infants; blood pressure control, coronary surgery, and transplants have increased the survival rate of adults. While life expectancy has been extended, however, more than 80 percent of those over age sixty-five have at least one chronic illness (Coile, 1986b).

Caring for Sicker People Longer. A patient saved from a heart attack will receive costly care for that episode of illness.

Living longer, the same patient may later have another heart attack or succumb to diseases that will consume additional resources. Patients with end-stage renal disease may receive kidney dialysis for years. A larger number of seriously disabled children are now being saved at birth, and they require substantial healthcare resources throughout their lives. We make no argument about the ethics of providing these services, but we do point out that both the use of healthcare services and the resulting costs are clearly increased when everyone's needs must be met.

Rapid Technological Change

Rapid changes in technology are affecting all healthcare organizations. Capabilities are increasing dramatically as highly technical and less invasive procedures proliferate. This growth is increasing capital costs, staffing costs, and training requirements, yet we are experiencing pressure to decrease costs through the use of DRGs and other prospective pricing systems. In this new era, we cannot assume that new technology will continue to be implemented or made accessible to patients at previous rates (Wilensky, 1988; Steinberg, 1985).

Major Construction Requirements and Costs

Requirements for facilities have changed substantially. For safety reasons, inpatient healthcare facilities are subject to more stringent and more frequently changing requirements than most other organizations are. Fire and safety codes are changed regularly, as new information becomes available. Similarly, changes in clinical practice and in customers' expectations also change facility-related requirements. Some of these changes cause existing buildings to fall out of compliance with the new codes, and functional facilities must be remodeled or replaced.

Facility and equipment changes entail substantial construction costs, at a time when reimbursements are shrinking. Because of the uncertainty of financial reimbursement and profitability, many healthcare organizations have also watched their credit ratings fall and their interest rates rise, which increases costs even more. In contrast, organizations that begin a transformation can improve their financial performance and their credit ratings.

The Trend Toward Health and Wellness

The American public has shown increased interest in wellness and in maintenance of health in general. Exercise, diet, and healthful behavior have helped reduce the risk of heart attack. The number of smokers in the United States has declined in tandem with the publicity given to the demonstrated health hazards of smoking. Today, smoking is banned in most public places and on airline flights. This trend, the result of changing social attitudes, is now being stressed by employers and insurance companies as a way to reduce direct healthcare costs. Higher premiums for life insurance are being charged to people who smoke; the higher rates reflect smokers' decreased life expectancy. We can expect similar variations in premiums for health insurance, based on documented life-style risk factors. This increased awareness of health is having an impact on both the type and the number of services needed and demanded (for example, there are now more sports-related injuries among adults).

The Changing Supply of Healthcare Professionals

The supply of healthcare professionals affects both the practice of medicine and the market costs of their skills. The demand for healthcare professionals changes along with technological and social changes.

Although there is debate about what the figures will be in the distant future, the supply of physicians (number per 1,000 population) is currently increasing for most specialties in the majority of U.S. metropolitan areas. By the end of 1990, there will be 2.80 physicians per 1,000 population, double the 1.40 per 1,000 in 1950 (Ginzberg, 1987). As a result of this increase, the base of patients is diminishing, along with the potential revenue per physician. Physicians are reacting to these developments by forming group practices, which offer better personal work schedules and lower overhead costs, and by diversifying to expand their bases of revenue. Many have chosen to compete with hospitals by offering such services as in-office X rays, diagnostic tests, and therapy.

At the same time, numbers of other healthcare professionals are declining in relation to demand. Nationally, there are shortages of registered nurses (particularly those with critical-care experience), physical therapists, occupational therapists, respiratory therapists, radiological technologists, and others. The shortages are most difficult for nonacute-care providers (such as nursing homes, home-care agencies, visiting nurse associations, and physicians' offices), third-party payers that use nurses and others as reviewers, and review agencies (such as professional review agencies and state and federal agencies). These shortages are driving up wages for nurses and others at a time when healthcare organizations can least afford such an expense. The shortages of allied health personnel are likely to continue during the next decade, until salaries, working conditions, and supplies of people have adjusted to the demands. This trend will continue as long as fewer students are entering allied health schools.

Most new technologies have introduced demands for specially trained physicians or new allied health professionals. Computed tomography (CT) scanning, magnetic resonance imaging (MRI), and other new technologies all require specially trained physicians and technicians. Thinking about coming changes in requirements for and availability of healthcare workers may help you plan more creatively and effectively and avoid recruitment problems.

> *Action Step*: **Carefully investigate skill-mix requirements, as well as reassignment of functions performed by professional staff to nonprofessional staff. Develop strong support services, and allow the professional staff to be more productive and effective. Make sure that reassignments are**

cost-effective. Develop effective retention plans, to reduce turnover.

Growth and Decline in Healthcare

Overall, healthcare is a growth industry, although acute-care hospitals are in the mature phase, and that portion has started to decline (Coile, 1986a). Healthcare revenues will continue to increase, in the range of 10 percent to 15 percent each year, at least until the year 2000. From 1975 to 1985, healthcare consistently outperformed all other industries, including communications (growth rate of 15.1 percent) and diversified services (15.8 percent). Much of this growth was fueled by advances in technology and by increases in the scope of services and in the average age of the population. In the past ten years, outpatient services have also grown dramatically, as less invasive technologies have been developed and treatment patterns have changed.

New technology is rapidly entering hospitals and other inpatient facilities; in acute inpatient care, however, market saturation has resulted from decreased use of acute-care inpatient services, excess capacity, displacement by other inpatient and outpatient services, technical maturity for many product lines, consumers' sophistication in purchase and use of services, and regulation (Ginzberg, 1987; Vraciu, 1985). Two current trends bear close monitoring: the aging of the population, and acquired immunodeficiency syndrome (AIDS). Unless more cost-effective inpatient and outpatient treatments are developed, these trends could dramatically increase the need for acute-care inpatient beds and many other services and facilities.

Each year, with fewer people admitted to hospitals, inpatient days are decreasing considerably. There were twelve million fewer inpatient days in each quarter of 1987 than there were in the first quarter of 1983, when patient days first began to decline. The decline in acute-care inpatient days has led to decreased occupancy and oversupply of hospital beds.

The tremendous pressure from business and industry to

hold down the cost of healthcare is due to the fact that the cost of American products is already high, and they have difficulty competing in the global marketplace. U.S. auto companies now state that healthcare adds more to the cost of a car than the price of steel does. In 1987, insurance costs for major employers went up an average of 20 percent, with some increases as high as 30 percent to 50 percent, and the National Manufacturers Association was reporting an average 30 percent increase in healthcare costs in 1988. Corporations also face an estimated $2 trillion liability in unfunded retiree healthcare costs. Tower, Perrin, Foster, and Crosby (cited in McManis, 1988, p. 31) estimate that if the U.S. automobile industry were to prefund these benefits, it would cost $39 billion, add $125 to the price of a car, and cut profits by 24 percent.

A serious threat to survival has been the shrinking profit margin experienced by hospitals. The average net patient margins dropped from 1.1 percent to 0.4 percent in 1987, following two consecutive years of decline. Total net margin was 4.9 percent, down from 5.5 percent in 1986. The continuing decline of profits will drive more hospitals, nursing homes, and other providers toward consolidation to remain in business (Gallivan, 1988).

Major Shift in the U.S. Economy

Although industrial and manufacturing organizations will continue to play a major role in the U.S. economy, there is a trend toward more information and service organizations (Ginzberg, 1987; Naisbitt, 1982). This generally means a shift toward smaller, more diversified, less unionized organizations. These organizations have tended to provide fewer healthcare benefits and benefits of other kinds. The smaller companies operate on smaller economic margins, and so less cash is available for benefits. Moreover, health and disability insurance and other benefits for individuals and small organizations are proportionately more costly than for larger organizations. The number of uninsured and underinsured people is estimated at over thirty million and growing rapidly. This places a major burden on healthcare organizations, businesses, and taxpayers.

Factors Influencing Healthcare Costs

Several competing factors exert pressure on healthcare costs, as illustrated in Figure 1. The value and impact of the different factors depend on interpretation of costs and benefits.

Interpretation of Costs and Benefits

People making decisions on healthcare policy and financing face dilemmas related to operational definitions and interpretations of costs and benefits, yet there is seldom clarification of these issues in publications or public debates. The following sections discuss some common and pressing questions.

What Is Included in Total Costs? Examples of costs that may or may not be included are hospitals, long-term-care facilities, home-care services, emergency services, ambulatory services, transportation, home care, time off work, child care, medications, and medical equipment. Consider this scenario: A patient receiving preadmission testing must take an extra day off work, drive several miles, pay for parking, and sometimes pay for child care and the tests. Should costs of the patient's time lost from work be included in the costs of medical care? Annual cost per capita now includes the costs of currently available technologies, which in the past were unavailable and were therefore not included in the cost per capita.

Costs to Whom? Virtually all payers consider their costs to be the only relevant costs. Each payer attempts to minimize its own out-of-pocket costs. An HMO's primary care physician receives a financial incentive for treating a patient with a back injury and preventing him or her from seeing an orthopedic physician or other specialized healthcare provider. Thus, the short-term out-of-pocket costs to the HMO or other payer are minimized. Nevertheless, if the HMO's physician does not have

Figure 1. Factors Influencing Healthcare Costs.

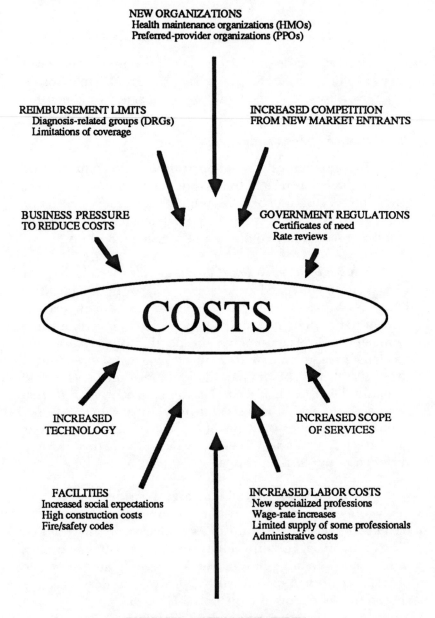

the skill to give effective treatment, the patient may remain off work and receive workers' compensation benefits for several weeks. The costs to the worker and to the employer's compensation plan are therefore larger but may not be considered.

Costs over What Denominator? Are we evaluating costs over a person's lifetime, costs per person per year, total costs per year for all patients, costs per medical episode, costs per inpatient stay, or costs per outpatient visit? This calculation can affect policy decisions. As an extreme example, consider the case of a patient who requires a kidney transplant. Costs per episode, costs during the next year, and costs during the person's remaining lifetime for the transplant may run to hundreds of thousands of dollars, but if the person returns to work and leads a productive life, there may be an offsetting financial contribution. The way we look at the cost-benefit relationship needs to be carefully analyzed.

How Are Benefits Calculated? A person has kidney failure and is placed on regular dialysis therapy. What is the benefit? That person's life is improved and extended, but how is the benefit calculated? This question is particularly difficult if the person is not working or contributing financially to society. Value decisions based on costs and benefits cannot be made without some explicit or implicit measure of benefit. How are value and cost-benefit ratio determined for public policy? There is no simple answer to these questions, yet they have a major impact on healthcare policy, healthcare available to patients, healthcare providers, and costs.

As a starting point, we suggest the following approach. Cost calculations should include all costs associated with an illness, even if only estimates are available. Thus, direct medical costs paid by the patient or any organization, costs of time off work, transportation expenses, and other costs to the patient should be included. If this approach is not used, the different payers make decisions to minimize their own costs by transferring costs to others, which increases total costs. Some measurement of benefit is necessary to settle issues of public policy. This is particularly important for chronic and lifelong conditions associated with AIDS, organ replacement, heart disease, mental illness, and muscular dystrophy.

Factors Increasing Costs

Increased Technology. Many costly high-technology services available today did not exist even as recently as 1965, when Medicare and Medicaid were implemented. Examples of such technology include the following:

- Advanced surgical procedures, including open-heart surgery, joint replacements, ear-bone implants, and cochlea implants
- Organ transplants, including kidney, heart, liver, lung, pancreas, and bone marrow
- Artificial organs, including hip joints, midear bones, and heart
- Testing equipment, including the CT scanner and MRI
- Noninvasive or less invasive treatment with arthroscopy, kidney and gallstone lithotripters, laser surgery, and gamma knives

Thus, healthcare and medicine today are far more advanced than they were twenty to thirty years ago. While the new healthcare capabilities have improved care and life expectancy, the cost has also been high.

Increased Scope of Services. Along with the increase in scope of services made available by technological advances, other services have also developed or expanded. Psychological counseling, social work services, occupational therapy, homecare services, and mobile testing services have all expanded capabilities and, in so doing, have increased costs.

Increased Acuity of Patients. Because of our increased knowledge and higher technology, we are able to prolong life;

therefore, the acuity level of inpatients and outpatients has increased. This, in turn, increases the sophistication, number, and cost of services. Skilled long-term-care facilities can now admit many patients who previously would have been admitted to acute-care hospitals, leaving hospitals to treat only the most acute patients. Other changes have contributed to this increased acuity level:

1. *Aging population*: Older people typically have more coexisting problems, recover less quickly, and require more care. For example, a patient who has gall bladder disease and needs surgery may also have diabetes and heart disease, which complicate care and recovery.
2. *Shifts in settings*: Many procedures have moved to ambulatory settings, leaving fewer but more acutely ill inpatients. Note that these changes have a host of implications for outpatient services and costs. To avoid a cost shift among payers, the total costs of inpatient and outpatient care must be considered..
3. *New technology*: Our technology allows us to prolong life with support systems, but these are very expensive in terms of labor and resources.

Increased Labor Costs. Total labor costs have increased, for three primary reasons: increased specialization, increased labor input for high-acuity patients, and wage increases (especially for professionals in short supply, such as nurses).

Technological advances, regulations, malpractice risk, and other factors have led organizations to use employees with higher credentials. Most other industries that are implementing new technologies also decrease their direct labor input; in hospitals, however, each new technology has required specially trained technicians, nurses, and physicians, and most such staffing needs are incremental.

Given the increased acuity of hospital inpatients, the ratio of nursing hours per inpatient day has risen. Resource requirements for pharmacists, physical therapists, and other healthcare professionals have also increased. Similar increases in acuity have been experienced in skilled-nursing facilities.

Wages are also higher. Between 1960 and 1980, wages for virtually all categories of staff were increased, to match wages for people with similar skills in other industries. Since about 1985, wages of nurses and other allied health providers have risen sharply. Because of shortages of these professionals, many healthcare organizations use staff from external agencies, a practice that further increases the costs of providing care. Unionization has also contributed to increased wages.

Administrative Costs. Administrative costs of healthcare organizations have increased out of proportion to costs for direct care. Staff members who fulfill the increased reimbursement and record-keeping requirements (preadmission certification, utilization review, billing), legal staff, and planning and marketing staff all increase administrative costs. Administrative costs related to insuring, providing, and reviewing healthcare in 1987 were estimated to be approximately 20 percent of total costs, or $100 billion (Ginzberg, 1987).

Institutionalization of More People. With increased life expectancy, improved medical care, and greater reliance on institutions in lieu of family support, more people are being institutionalized. This trend, along with limited reimbursement, has caused a shortage of long-term-care facilities for disabled and elderly people. This shortage will continue as the elderly population increases, unless reimbursement is also increased to the point where new facilities will be financially viable.

Time and Cost to Gain Approval of Services and Products. It takes several years of laboratory tests and clinical trials to gain approval for new healthcare services and products. The Federal Drug Administration requires years of testing, which costs millions of dollars and delays treatment with new drugs. Clearly, there is a trade-off between the costs of early release and the costs of continued testing. A recent exception was made with the release of a drug earlier than scheduled to treat AIDS patients, since AIDS patients die without treatment.

Factors Decreasing Costs

Government and Business Pressure to Reduce Costs. For several years, the federal government, state governments, business and industrial organizations, and third-party payers simply absorbed or passed on increased costs to the people who purchased their products or paid their expenses. In the face of rapidly rising costs, government and business organizations have expressed major concern and have assumed a much stronger role in the healthcare industry. Although a number of different approaches have been attempted, it is difficult to document whether they actually have reduced costs. Examples include federal and state laws and regulations (such as those involving certificates of need), reimbursement limits for services covered and amounts paid, business and union participation in healthcare planning and review, and promotion of competitive bidding to provide healthcare services.

New Organizations. New types of organizations have developed in response to demands from business for more predictable, controllable, and lower healthcare costs. Substantial numbers of HMOs and PPOs have developed and are offered as options to employees. These plans compete, on the basis of services and costs, with traditional insurance plans. Their market penetration varies widely but is increasing. HMOs, while effective in reducing hospital costs, often increase outpatient costs.

> *Action Step*: **Implement processes to continually improve quality, and develop quantitative measures of the processes and outcomes of medical care and healthcare. Without such measures, third-party payers, businesses, and patients will**

continue to make their decisions on the basis of price alone.

The competitive marketplace has also caused tremendous moral and ethical conflicts for healthcare executives. What we are seeing are medical "arms races," with a narrow focus on cost control and profitability that, in the long run, may be counterproductive.

External Planning and Marketing Efforts

In today's environment, passively waiting for patients to arrive no longer works. The competitive environment requires a much better understanding of your customers, your customers' requirements, your capabilities, and how you plan to change. Planning and marketing efforts should be an essential part of your organization. These efforts must involve far more sophistication than simply running advertisements. New, computerized data bases cross-index healthcare use with demographic factors by zip code or census tract, so that an organization can predict the likely demand for specific services in specific areas.

Closure and Restructuring to Provide Services

Because of decreases in use of inpatient facilities, new reimbursement restrictions, and cost increases, unprecedented numbers of hospitals are closing or being absorbed by acquisitions and mergers. Several forms of corporate restructuring are leading to both internal and external environmental changes, such as corporate reorganization of hospitals, joint ventures, consolidations, and networking.

Diversification

The scope of the healthcare industry is changing dramatically through diversification activities. The three primary types of diversification are as follows:

1. *Healthcare diversification:* Hospitals, long-term-care facilities, physicians' groups, and so on are diversifying into patient services, functions, and resources not traditionally provided. For example, hospitals are opening rehabilitation units, adding home-care and medical equipment divisions, and opening ambulatory clinics in shopping malls. A complete categorization, or taxonomy, of healthcare services is provided in Chapter Five.

2. *Geographical diversification:* Large hospitals and group practices have begun to diversify into nontraditional geographical settings. Diversification typically includes satellite ambulatory-care centers surrounding a hospital or a physicians' group practice. Some organizations go on to diversify even more. For example, both the Cleveland Clinic, in Ohio, and the Mayo Clinic, in Minnesota, have opened healthcare facilities in Florida. Kaiser, which began in California, currently has facilities in several states.

3. *Nonhealthcare diversification:* Hospitals, in particular, have been diversifying into many nonhealthcare endeavors, usually through for-profit subsidiaries. A day-care center, for example, allows an organization to attract and keep employees who have had problems finding day care for their children. Other ventures include hotels, shopping centers, computer stores, landscaping, fast-food outlets, and real-estate holdings (such as office and apartment buildings). The purpose of these for-profit corporations is to generate capital, which can then be used for health-related projects at the discretion of the holding company's board, without being used as a direct offset to payments by third-party payers.

Legal Liability and Malpractice Risk

Legal liability and malpractice risk have become serious environmental factors and have influenced the practice patterns and organization of healthcare resources. Jury Verdict Research of Solon, Ohio, reported that the mean malpractice settlement was $367,319 in 1979 and $962,258 in 1982 (Raske

and Eisenman, 1986), and settlements have been steadily increasing. The cost of malpractice insurance for some surgeons
practicing near metropolitan areas now exceeds $75,000 per
year. As a result, some physicians refuse to care for high-risk
populations; for example, the number of obstetricians has
fallen. Another common response is to develop a large-volume
group practice, where risks can be shared.

Reimbursement and Cost Control

Many different varieties of reimbursement and cost control have to exist. Almost every insurance company, HMO, PPO,
state agency, federal agency, and employer has multiple contracts, each with unique restrictions on services, reimbursement, costs, patient deductibles, and so on. Internal cost
controls are being implemented in virtually all healthcare organizations as a means of remaining competitive, developing new
programs, and developing capital for facility and equipment
changes.

Changing Expectations of Employees

To allow employees to achieve their full potential, we must
involve them in identifying problems and developing improvements. Strong desire to maintain the status quo will make some
employees suspicious of new programs and other changes.
Nevertheless, employees in all industries, especially professionals, expect greater involvement in decision making. We must
allow physicians, nurses, pharmacists, and other professional
and nonprofessional groups to participate in decisions that
affect them if we expect them to perform to their full capacity. A
new openness must prevail in management.

Management Information Systems

In this competitive, reimbursement-restricted, and
rapidly changing environment, management information is
crucial to informed, correct decisions. One key challenge is to

develop systems that effectively address our rapidly increasing information requirements. Without improvements in information processing, labor costs increase. Improved systems for processing information are needed in many areas, including cost determination, clinical management of cases (such as in utilization review), performance planning and monitoring, quality planning and monitoring, reimbursement management, medical record management (particularly with geographically dispersed facilities), and patient service management (for waiting times, service times, and information for patients).

Board Pressure on Executives

Given the magnitude of these environmental changes, as well as the implications of their social and financial impact on healthcare organizations, boards of directors are placing more pressure on executives to meet difficult and often conflicting goals. Executives are expected to provide the latest technology, competitive prices, high-quality services, and more access to services, as well as profits.

When financial or other problems occur, a board often decides that the executive is at fault, and the executive is fired, justly or not. In some areas of the United States, executive turnover is higher than 30 percent per year. Boards should be educated regularly about the changing healthcare environment, as well as about the trends of their organizations' operations.

Implications for Healthcare Management

What are the implications of these environmental changes for leaders in the healthcare industry? In particular, what are the implications for *you?* The leaders of healthcare organizations must anticipate, initiate, and sponsor change. In essence, you must become a change agent. Your continued success will depend on your finding trade-offs among the conflicting goals and requirements of your many customers. You must also recognize that this is risky business. Most large organizations tend to drive out or silence change agents. Later in this

Figure 2. Product Profitability Curve.

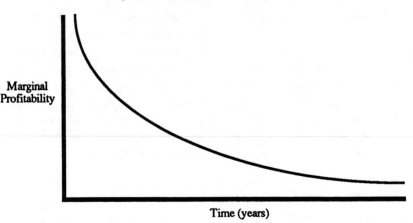

book, we will discuss approaches to increasing organizational readiness for change and creating a support system for change agents.

Product Profitability and Innovation Strategy. Your strategy will depend on where the services and products offered by your organization are in their respective product lives. Healthcare services and products, like other services and products, tend to follow a profitability curve, as illustrated in Figure 2. Shortly after a new product or service is developed and refined for general sale, its marginal profitability is highest. This is because the product or service is unique, unavailable from other organizations. In fact, many products are protected by patents for seventeen years. This initial high return is used to recover the high costs of developing and promoting a new product or service. As the years pass, however, many other organizations begin to offer competing services or products, and marginal profitability falls.

Two extremes of management strategies related to innovation during the life of a product or a service are as follows:

1. *Maximize innovation of new services and products*: This strategy works best in academic health centers and large medical

centers, which have the ability and resources to develop new services and strategies. New and highly specialized services, such as lithotripter procedures to break up kidney stones, laser surgery on eyes, and highly technical kinds of drug administration after heart attacks, are examples of new services and products. In organizations offering such high-technology services, the primary focus should be on innovation and creativity for new products and services.

2. *Minimize costs on well-established services and products*: This strategy works best in smaller hospitals, which have limited new technology but also lower costs. In these organizations, the primary focus should be on innovation to reduce costs and increase the volume of services.

The challenge in every organization is to maintain a scope of services acceptable to its customers and simultaneously maintain financial viability. Services and products should be reevaluated periodically, so that their continued value can be determined.

Market Recognition. Confusion is consumers' usual reaction to the variety of healthcare options. They are faced with advertisements by healthcare plans with similar names and coverages, advertisements by hospitals with similar services, complex limitations and forms for healthcare reimbursement, and mixed information about quality and other characteristics. To compete effectively, healthcare organizations must establish market recognition of their services and products. Market recognition is best established through provision of high quality and value to customers. A well-trained marketing plan is also useful in planning and communicating your organization's services and products. Nevertheless, marketing and advertising cannot match the benefits of word-of-mouth advertising by satisfied customers.

Summary

This chapter has provided a brief overview of the complicated environment facing healthcare organizations. Now more than ever, with unprecedented changes in both the external and the internal environments, strong leadership is necessary. Your organization cannot compete effectively by using traditional kinds of response to change. Given the broadness of the issues, rapidly developing new technologies, changing expectations, and increasing risks, you will need to develop strategies that use collaborative input into decision making and implementation.

Avoid the way that some healthcare organizations plan, which reminds us of a passage from *Alice's Adventures in Wonderland* (Carroll, 1921, p. 89):

> "Would you tell me, please, which way I ought to go from here?"
>
> "That depends a good deal on where you want to get to," said the [Cheshire] Cat.
>
> "I don't much care where—" said Alice.
>
> "Then it doesn't matter which way you go," said the Cat.

A lack of vision or direction can keep us running faster just to stay in place—or we may even lose ground. The solution is to think about how to align and involve your board, administration, medical staff, and employees in the transformation of your organization.

Chapter Three

❧❦❧

Anticipating and Adapting to Changing Requirements

As we have said before, one critically important characteristic of successful leaders is their ability to anticipate, adapt to, and manage change. Daryl Conner, a leading advocate of managing change, states, "The capacity to manage fundamental, traumatic change will be a critical distinction between winners and losers in the future" (Greene, 1988, p. 20). Transformation of the organization will not occur unless leaders recognize the need to manage change.

One conceptual framework for transformational leadership views transformation as a three-act drama, as illustrated in Figure 3. According to Tichy and Devanna (1986a, pp. 28, 30), "The need for change is triggered by environmental pressures. But not all organizations respond to signals from the environment indicating change. The external trigger event must be perceived and responded to by leaders in the first phase of the transformation process." The transformational leader focuses attention on the transformation of the business from its current state to a better one. Figure 3 emphasizes the importance of a leader as a change sponsor and change agent.

Healthcare leaders must recognize that any major change affecting the healthcare industry is likely to affect their organizations. This is why scanning the environment is a critical skill.

For a change to be implemented, everyone involved must endorse it. Rosabeth Moss Kanter, Harvard Business School professor and author of *The Change Masters*, has said that organizations will not achieve the desired results unless employees understand the need for change and accept individual responsibility for implementing it. According to Kanter, "If people start

41

Figure 3. Tichy and Devanna Transformational Leader Framework.

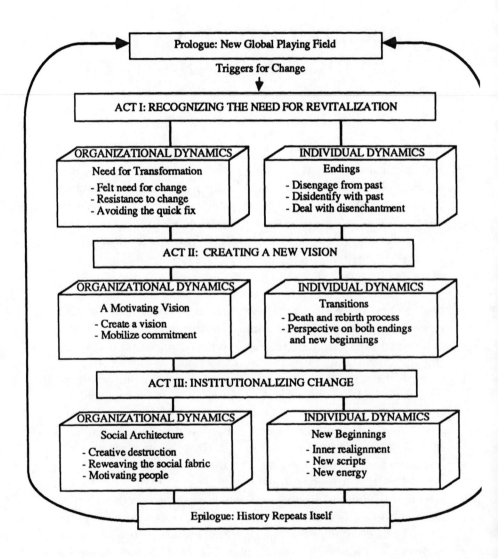

Source: Tichy and Devanna, 1986a, p. 29. Reprinted with permission.

to say, 'This isn't my job' or 'It's not my fault; it's their fault,' then no one accepts responsibility and nothing gets accomplished" (cited in Greene, 1988, p. 26).

Methods of Anticipating Change

The stimulus for most major changes in healthcare institutions is found in the outside environment. Some examples may help clarify this statement. Major reimbursement changes have been developed by third-party payers. These changes include the use of diagnosis-related groups (DRGs), the requirement to obtain a second physician's opinion concerning the need for surgery, restrictions on payments for some services, and managed-care contracts. Other stimuli found outside healthcare institutions include changing demographics, changing family responsibilities (due in part to dual-career families), changing construction and safety codes, changing attitudes about quality of life that lead to health-and-wellness practices in the population, and changing availability of healthcare professionals.

> *Action Step*: **Be proactive. Carefully study the environment external to your organization, to predict potential trends and changes and develop strategies to deal with them.**

To predict change and develop strategies, you need to consider several types of information, as shown in Figure 4. Sources of this information, methods of obtaining it, integration of the information into a vision for the future, and evaluation of change actions should then be considered.

> *Action Step*: **Teach your management staff how to survey the external environment for signs of change that may affect healthcare and your organization. Monitor trends and new developments, and discuss them at staff meetings. Explore ways to become more proactive.**

Figure 4. Types of Information for Predicting Changes.

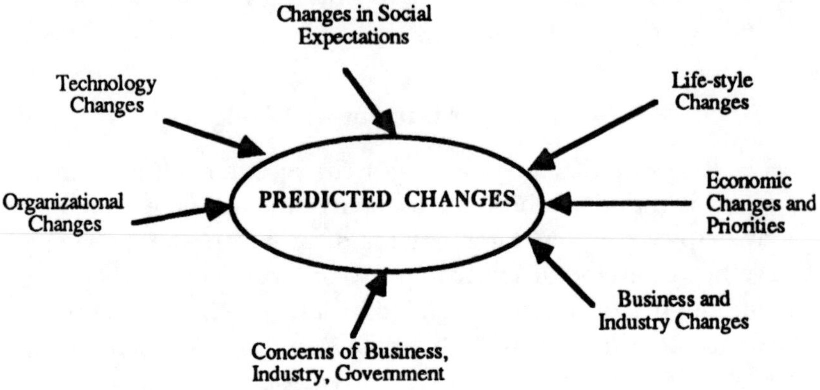

Changes in Social
Expectations

Technology
Changes

Life-style
Changes

Organizational
Changes

PREDICTED CHANGES

Economic
Changes and
Priorities

Concerns of Business,
Industry, Government

Business and
Industry Changes

Using Different Types of Information

Several different types of information can help you fore-cast and understand potential changes.

Changes in Social Expectations. Changes in what people expect in the way of services, waiting times, confidentiality, and respect, not to mention amenities, change the way we design facilities and provide services to patients. For example, patients no longer accept long waits to see by a physician. More con-sumers expect and demand responsive providers, as well as a high level of amenities. A second example of changing social expectations and life-styles concerns dual career families. When there is no one at home to care for elderly parents and other relatives, there are increasing demands for long-term-care facili-ties and home-care services. A third example involves customers' growing sophistication, which entails the expectation that healthcare professionals will provide better information. This change is positive because informed patients (and their fami-lies) can become more involved in treatment and learn how to provide care for themselves and others at home.

Life-Style Changes. Such long-standing habits as smoking and alcohol consumption have caused respiratory, heart, and liver disease. The current trends to decrease smoking, alcohol consumption, and cholesterol intake and to increase exercise have already lowered the rates of respiratory and heart disease. Recent information on the harmful effects of sunbathing has changed the notion that a "bronzed" skin is healthy.

Economic Changes and Priorities. The priority given to healthcare expenses relative to other public and private expenditures will affect both the types and the quantities of healthcare services that people demand. In periods of economic depression, for example, expenditures for many healthcare services go down.

Changes Implemented by U.S. and Foreign Business and Industry. Changes in the healthcare industry tend to follow similar changes in other industries by five or ten years. Reviewing major industrial changes may help you predict future changes in the healthcare industry. For example, consider the cost-reduction focus of industry during the 1970s, which hospitals implemented during the 1980s, or the total-quality focus that industry initiated about 1980 and that hospitals are now beginning to use.

Many major corporations are reducing the number of their suppliers, as a way of improving quality and reducing costs. They ask their suppliers to demonstrate quality-improvement processes and quality-control processes in order to continue as suppliers. Therefore, we can expect corporations like Ford Motor Company to reduce the number of their healthcare suppliers soon and to require suppliers to demonstrate quality-improvement processes.

Concerns of Business and Industry. When industry leaders voice concern about healthcare costs, you can expect their involvement in a variety of cost-containment initiatives. This is especially true in geographical areas that are dominated by a few large industrial and business organizations.

Mergers, Corporate Reorganization, and Diversification. Organizational changes inside and outside the healthcare industry are likely to affect your organization. For example, the merger of two industrial organizations with different insurance or health maintenance organizations can radically affect coverage of healthcare services, prices, and decisions about which health-care providers will be used, especially within a geographical area.

Types of corporate reorganization occurring in the healthcare industry include joint ventures, consolidations, and networks formed among providers to capture market share and limit consumers' use of competitors' services.

Most large healthcare organizations, to varying degrees, have implemented three types of diversification: healthcare di-versification, to offer a broader range of services and products; geographical diversification, to capture market share; and non-healthcare diversification, to generate additional revenue. Orga-nizational changes within the healthcare industry should be monitored carefully, since they can have a large and immediate impact on your own organization.

Technological Developments in Healthcare. These new de-velopments will affect service demands, facilities, equipment, staff, and costs. For example, the introduction of laser surgery and other technological improvements into hospitals has vir-tually eliminated hospital stays for ophthalmology patients.

Availability of Healthcare Professionals and Resources. The supply, skills, and cost of physicians, nurses, laboratory techni-cians, physical therapists, and other healthcare professionals affect the delivery and cost of healthcare services and products. Similarly, the availability of other resources (like land, facilities, equipment, and money) also affects an organization's ability to change.

Locating Sources of Information

There are many sources of information and many ways to identify changes in the external market. Useful sources of information can be found both within and outside your organization. The following sections describe such sources.

External Customers. Peters (1987, p. 176) recommends becoming obsessed with listening: "Become 'transparent' to (that is, listen to) customers — end users, reps, distributors, franchisees, retailers, suppliers. Listen frequently. Listen systematically — and unsystematically. Listen for facts — and for perceptions. Listen 'naively.' Use as many listening techniques as we can conjure up." Regularly ask your patients, referring physicians, and other external customers to tell you about their requirements, needs, and the changes they expect in their practices or life-styles. Customers are particularly valuable in helping you forecast evolutionary changes in products and services. For revolutionary change, however, customers normally cannot predict change. For example, healthcare customers could not have predicted technologies like kidney dialysis, CT scanners, or lasers. These technologies were developed by physicians and manufacturers to meet professionally identified needs for less invasive diagnosis and therapy.

Sometimes it makes sense to be in the lead, but not in first place. If you are too far in the lead, your customers may not understand or appreciate the changes you make. Therefore, they may not use a new service or product. Likewise, your board members, physicians, and employees may not understand rapid changes. It is management's responsibility to educate everyone involved, at an appropriate rate, so that people can fulfill their roles.

Business Leaders. Healthcare leaders should regularly meet with local leaders of large and small businesses. These leaders and their organizations are major buyers of healthcare insurance and services. Understanding their unique problems will help you tailor (and, perhaps, price) your services.

Business Publications. It is wise to scan popular and business publications, such as *Boardroom, Business Week,* Crain's business newspapers, *Fortune, Newsweek, Time,* and the *Wall Street*

Journal. For top healthcare executives, these publications may be more important than healthcare publications.

Scientific Publications. These are useful in predicting technological changes, particularly those of a revolutionary nature.

Conferences. Attending conferences for business and healthcare leaders will give you insights into the local and national issues that affect healthcare.

> *Action Step*: **Teach your managers what to look for, how to report information, and how to develop a plan for the future. Allow them to make valuable community contacts.**

Professional Associations for Business. In addition to those specifically for the healthcare industry, business associations — for example, the American Management Association, business "round tables," and so forth — can provide a much broader understanding of business's concerns.

Forecasting Books, Services, and Consultants. These sources predict a wide variety of changes, but you must determine the likelihood that these changes will affect the healthcare industry.

Federal and State Agencies. Pay special attention to government agencies that provide direct or indirect funding for healthcare services, education, and research.

Healthcare Publications. Some of these predict or report on changes in the industry. Ask managers and supervisors to determine key points of articles and discuss them at monthly staff meetings. The objective is to make people stretch and think more strategically.

Other Healthcare Institutions. You can learn from other organizations, including your competitors. Find the very best example of each service or product, and determine how the organization has achieved its performance. Practice by discovering the best features of comparable services or products all over the world. For example, if you find that a hospital or other healthcare organization is succeeding with a new approach, your organization may be able to design and implement a service to meet some need before your competitors do.

Consumers. People in the community are an important source of information about your current services, changes occurring in your area, and potential demand for modification of your services and products.

> *Action Step*: **Regularly share articles found by anyone on your staff, or designate someone to extract articles from the publications you do not regularly read, and circulate them.**

Internal Sources. Your staff is an important source of ideas because staff members should have up-to-date information on technological and other changes affecting their professions. Internal sources of information about external changes include board members, physicians, nurses, and other professionals. Board members bring both internal and external views, since they are often external business leaders as well. Physicians are important sources of information about change, especially physicians who conduct research or work with large national organizations. Success in research can help your organization change early and achieve success in a research-related area. Internal sources are most likely to contribute information in areas affecting clinical care, technology, patient services and products, and management approaches.

Obtaining Information

You should use several different methods or sources to obtain information, since no one method or source is best for every situation.

Personal Meetings. Direct, personal conversations with customers, business representatives, and others are very valuable because they allow two-way communication. Have such conversations with external sources several times per month. Professional meetings are another good approach because you can see many people at the same time.

Telephone Conversations. These also allow two-way communication, but unless you know the person well, he or she may not speak candidly.

Survey Questionnaires. These are most useful in quantifying customers' perceptions, but they should be used in addition to personal conversations.

Study of Competitors' Statistics. These can be assembled from many sources, including the American Hospital Association, your state hospital association, the Health Care Finance Administration (for hospitals providing care to Medicare patients), and state agencies. Medicare cost reports filed by hospitals are subject to the Freedom of Information Act and can be obtained through the Medicare intermediary. There is a delay and a charge, but the information is available. The goal is to know as much as possible about your competitors.

Union Contract Negotiations. Much information related to healthcare issues can be gathered during contract negotiations at large corporations. Once a contract is final, it also provides specific information about healthcare reimbursement and coverage, information helpful in predicting future demands for healthcare services and products.

Review Organizations. Review organizations are a good source of information about potential changes. The Health Care Finance Administration and the Joint Commission on Accreditation of Healthcare Organizations publish documents and reports on current topics in research and development.

Legislative Updates. Proposed and pending legislation can provide valuable information. Regular communication with legislators can give you lead time to initiate changes, besides allowing you input into the legislative process. Regulatory-compliance reports and other government publications are also sources of useful information.

Integrating Information into a Vision for the Future

Integration of information from diverse sources is necessary for separating major changes and trends from unrelated and possibly irrelevant events. The goal is to look at things over time, and one simple but very useful approach is to graph the relevant data. An understanding of variations in processes is very important to asking appropriate questions and making correct decisions. Evaluating a graph of data over time, as opposed to looking at a measurement from a single point in time, allows you to separate unique events from normal variations. Deming (1986) refers to the unique event as a "special cause" of variation, and to normal variations as "common causes" of variation.

Integration of information requires, first, synthesis of information from diverse sources and, next, a search for logical patterns. For example, if many businesses in an area are experiencing unacceptable problems with substance abuse among employees, then there is a likely market for substance-abuse services. If the federal government is working on DRG (diagnosis-related groups)-based research related to physicians' services, then a combined DRG payment for the hospital and physicians is a potential change. Answering the following types of questions may be helpful in integrating information into a vision for the future:

- What opinions are major industrial and business leaders offering?
- Are several business leaders from the same industry offering similar opinions? From different industries?

- Are patients and other customers expressing similar concerns?
- Is there a correlation between the opinions and proposed actions of large corporations and federal or state agencies?
- Are there logical actions that fit several of the circumstances being observed?
- Are corporations implementing new management processes that may be useful in healthcare?
- What new approaches are being taken in other healthcare organizations?

Evaluating Alternative Actions for Change

Once you have a vision of the future, the next step is to develop and evaluate the potential alternatives for action available to your organization. All healthcare organizations face limitations of staff, money, and other resources; you cannot pursue all the alternatives. The idea is to select a few important issues that will have a major effect on your organization. Essentially, you and your decision-support staff should simulate the marketing, operational, financial, and other impacts of different alternatives. Your actions will also be based on your assumptions about what your competitors are doing.

One useful approach is to evaluate a number of alternatives or scenarios, using different criteria. Begin by identifying all the relevant criteria (such as estimated profitability, quality improvement, contribution to image, and referrals to other services); there should be several different ones. Table 3 is limited to three criteria, for purposes of illustration. The relative importance of each criterion should be given a weight, as illustrated in the table. Each potential alternative is then listed, and its relative contribution to each criterion is estimated. To calculate the weighted score for each criterion, multiply its relative contribution by the relative weight. Weighted scores can then be summed for each alternative, to indicate each one's relative merit. In this process, group members often calculate the weights individually at first, so that members will not influence one another. Then it is helpful to display all the weights, discuss

Table 3. Evaluation Matrix for Alternatives.

	Criterion 1: Profit	Criterion 2: Quality	Criterion 3: Referrals	Total
Relative weight	8	9	6	
Alternative 1: Referral service	7	2	10	
Weighted score	56	18	60	134
Alternative 2: Commercial store	9	2	3	
Weighted score	72	18	18	108
Alternative 3: Improved communication	4	9	6	
Weighted score	32	81	36	149

them, and come to an agreement on relative weights and relative contributions of the alternatives. The impacts of various alternatives can also be simulated for different predictions of change, in order to select the best alternative. Those with the highest scores are then investigated in more detail. It is important to remember that this is a tool to help in understanding the alternatives. It will not yield exact results, but it does provide a way of reducing the number of the alternatives you will investigate in detail. Another important benefit of this approach is that the discussions that it calls for help people understand the variables involved, as well as the values and goals of the organization.

The Threshold of Corporate Change

Leaders must create a vision for change, communicate this vision to others in the organization, and motivate people in the organization to accomplish the change. Nevertheless, we feel that there is a limit to the rate of change that an organization can tolerate, and we will call this limit the *threshold of corporate change*. Beyond the threshold, the organization becomes dysfunctional; its leader may even be fired. The goal is learning to make improvements as rapidly as possible, without exceeding the threshold of corporate change.

Every person and every organization has a threshold of change. It cannot be specifically calculated, but the smaller the organization, the more likely it is to endure a rapid rate of change, provided that the leaders are consistent in their vision and communications. Large organizations tend to have long-standing cultures entrenched in the past and low thresholds of change.

Although an organization may have an overall tolerance of change, its threshold will depend on the proposed change, the way the mission is crafted, and the buy-in achieved among affected parties. Changes consistent with the corporate culture and vision will have a higher threshold than changes contrary to the corporate culture and perceived as arbitrary.

Determining the Threshold of Change

Since, as we have said, corporate culture involves behavior patterns, beliefs, and many other factors, changing the culture of an organization often means changing employees' beliefs and attitudes. Different approaches are possible in determining the approximate threshold of corporate change; the following are suggested.

Understand the Corporate Culture. First, you must try to understand the culture of your organization. How difficult or easy has it been to implement change in the past? What was the most dramatic change during the last ten years? How did people in the organization react to that change? What things reduced resistance, and what things increased resistance to change?

Understand the Current Situation. The more comfortable the current situation, the less willing people will be to undertake any change. If, for example, a physicians' group practice has been profitable for years, the threshold for change is likely to be low. Change represents a risk, whereas the current situation appears relatively free of risk. By contrast, if a nursing home has been losing large sums of money and is on the verge of bankruptcy, leaders and employees may tolerate a major change because maintaining the status quo is liable to lead to bankruptcy and unemployment.

Determine People's Positions on the Proposed Change. The position and relative strength of each person or group should be estimated in relation to a proposed change. A simple approach is to view each person's position with respect to the change on a scale of − 10 through + 10, with − 10 meaning "strongly opposed" and + 10 meaning "strongly in favor." In general, a person cannot be moved more than a couple of points along this scale during any presentation or any month, and any attempt to hurry movement will result in failure. It takes time for a person to understand and accept a proposed change. Scores for individuals can be grouped, as a way of measuring a department's or an organization's position on a proposed change. This simple approach can be used by any manager. More sophisticated approaches are also available, but they require more knowledge and resources. A similar method, known as *force-field analysis*, lists driving forces and restraining forces opposite each other, indicating the relative strength of each (GOAL/QPC, 1988).

Measure Resistance to Change. Resistance to a specific change can be measured. O.D. Resources, Inc. (1988), offers a scale that measures individual resistance to a proposed change. Each of twenty-five factors is ranked on a scale of 1 to 10, with 1 indicating the least resistance. Results can be summarized for each of the twenty-five factors. They can also be expressed cumulatively, to provide management an understanding of the resistance.

By integrating knowledge about your corporate culture, your current situation, current positions on a proposed change, and resistance, you can estimate your organization's threshold of change. You can then plan how to present proposed changes at a rate that will make support for them more likely.

Raising the Threshold of Change

The threshold of change can be raised, but this takes time and effort. The threshold depends on confidence in leaders, as well as on one's own personal sense of risk. The following approaches can be used to raise the threshold of change.

Demonstrate Leadership. Your commitment to the change must be evident. If the leader is not trusted or perceived as committed, there will be a low threshold of change.

Convey the Need and Purpose for Change. The need for any change must be made clear. Because it is easier not to change, people must sense some need for change. The purpose of the change should also be communicated. How are the organization and individuals going to benefit? For example, must the waiting time in outpatient services be reduced because patients are complaining and going to a competitor?

Involve People in Change. Communicate regularly about the change, its purpose, and its expected benefits. Involve staff people in planning the change. Their involvement will lead to understanding, ownership, and support in implementation, provided that the change is appropriate.

Reduce Personal Risk. The threshold of change will be raised as people perceive less personal threat. If someone feels sure of continuing to have a meaningful job or role in the organization, then he or she will be more supportive of change. Job security and maintenance of social relations are important to raising the threshold of change. Applaud improvements, rather than asking why changes were not made sooner. You must protect, compliment, and reward those who work to make improvements.

Develop a Record of Successful Changes. As people see a series of successful small changes, their fear of change will diminish, and their support of future changes will increase. Success raises the threshold of change for the future.

Components of Transformation

The transformation of an organization has nine vital components. We will introduce the components here; subse-

Figure 5. Components of Transformation.

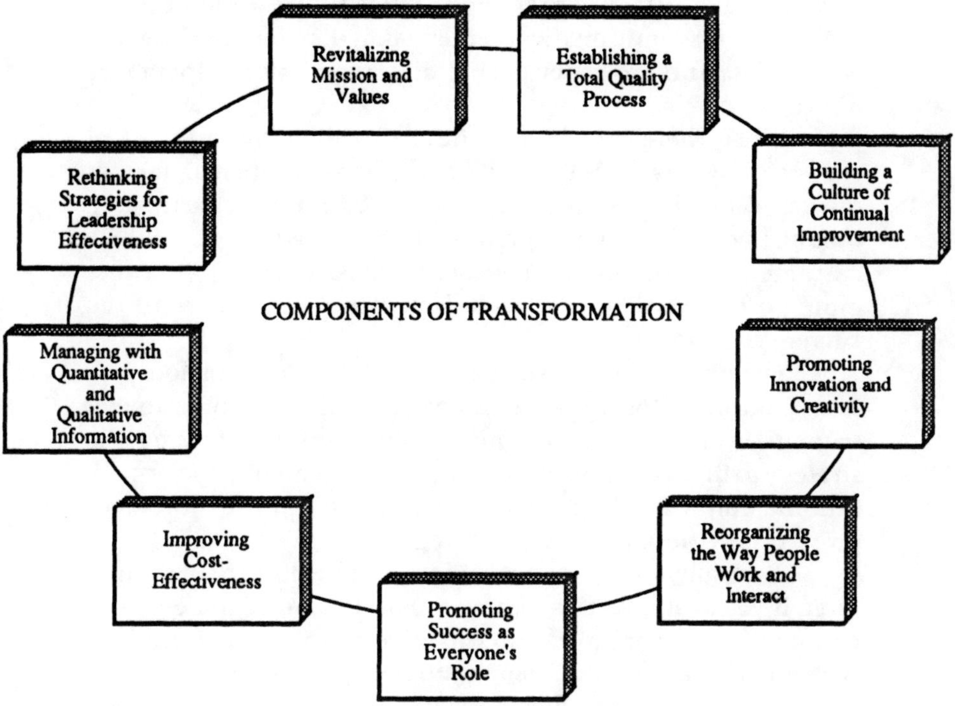

quent chapters provide more detail on how to accomplish a transformation. Action may be initiated and may progress at different rates for each of the nine components, but they are illustrated together in Figure 5.

Why Change?

Probably the most basic question for healthcare executives is "Why change?" We have been successful in the past doing the same things; why change course now? The same questions are asked frequently by most middle managers, who are not as aware as top managers are of the sweeping environmental changes affecting all healthcare organizations. This attitude toward change is also prevalent in healthcare organizations (especially academic medical centers) that have remained profitable to date and are experiencing high inpatient occupancy or utilization levels.

Since there is a human desire to limit the amount of change, why change? The majority of environmental factors discussed in Chapter Two imply a bleak future for healthcare organizations that fail to understand their customers and their customers' needs, fail to meet those needs, and fail to become more cost-effective and provide innovative alternatives to the current situation.

Healthcare executives generally follow one of four options: ignoring the organizational culture and environment; managing around the organizational culture; changing the strategy to fit the organizational culture; or changing the organizational culture to fit the strategy. The last option is the best, given solid vision, goals, and strategy.

Basically, you have two choices as a healthcare executive. First, if you avoid the risk of being proactive, you can be almost certain that your organization will fall prey to the organizations that do change to meet their customers' requirements. Executives in organizations that wait and see are likely to be left behind in a competitive environment and may lose their jobs. Second, you can begin transforming your organizations, realizing that some of the changes that you attempt may fail. Executives who begin transformations do court high risks, but they may be able to position their organizations and themselves to compete more effectively and lead the industry. By maintaining close communication with customers, suppliers, and employees, you lower your risks.

No matter which path you choose, there is no question that you face risk. If you want to avoid risk, you should find another occupation, because healthcare management has become a high-risk business.

Revitalizing Mission and Values

The first important step in the transformation process is to review and revitalize the mission and values of your organization, using your vision for the organization as your guide. Almost every hospital and healthcare organization has a written mission statement; such statements are usually long, formal, all-encompassing, and very vague, with little meaning for employees or external customers. If your organization is like most, your mission statement attempts to promise all things to all people at all times.

The mission statement should be simple, couched in terms that are easily understood by all. In addition to the statement of mission, simple statements of the organization's values are also important, so that employees can identify with the goals of the organization and see their roles within the whole.

Well-defined statements of mission and values are essential to using the other components of transformation effectively. You cannot move people in a common direction if you do not say where you are going. Here is an example of a simple mission statement: "Memorial Medical Center will be a regional leader in providing state-of-the-art healthcare services and products to meet the needs of our customers. Our goal is to continually improve services and products for our customers, allowing us to remain profitable." Each organization must develop statements uniquely suited to its environment, customers, and goals.

If you define your mission and values in terms that all employees understand and support, then specific policies and procedures become less important. Without understandable missions and values, managers must try to address each of many possible circumstances with a unique policy or procedure, each of which consumes substantial resources and tends to limit the creativity of employees by posing numerous limitations.

Obtaining comments directly from employees is very useful in developing values statements. Collectively, employees embody the corporate culture, and they will be the people who live out the new values.

Establishing a Total Quality Process

The total quality process is the primary theme of transformation to achieve organizational success. Quality is becoming the focal point of many successful U.S. industries and will be the focus of U.S. healthcare during the 1990s.

Hospitals and other healthcare organizations have been evaluating quality for years — or have they? Healthcare providers have traditionally defined the term *quality* in a very narrow sense, focusing almost entirely on measures of the structure, process, and, more recently, outcomes of the clinical services provided. These are certainly measures of quality, but they are only part of the total quality approach, which includes meeting the product and service requirements of all internal and external customers. *Customer* is a general term used to refer to any person or organization that receives a service, a product, or information from another. The person or organization providing the service, product, or information is referred to as the *supplier*.

The quality situation for healthcare organizations is complicated by the unique functions that physicians serve. Physicians admit patients and order the tests, procedures, and supplies provided by a hospital, nursing home, or other healthcare organization. Hence, they are customers, in one sense, because they choose the institution and determine the types and volumes of products and services provided. Physicians are also suppliers because they provide services directly to patients. The patients and their families are customers in the sense that they receive the products and services and make judgments about whether to return or refer others to the healthcare organization. Moreover, there is an additional set of customers to consider: people with whom you work every day, for whom services are provided, and from whom services are received. People are both suppliers and customers at different times.

Quality and value will be very important in the future. As healthcare costs continue to escalate, federal and state government (through Medicare, Medicaid, and other programs), health maintenance organizations, preferred-provider organizations, third-party payers, employers, and employee groups (such as unions) will make comparisons among healthcare providers. Customers will compare costs and measures of quality and value in making decisions about which organizations will be reimbursed for providing healthcare services and products to their customers and employees. The question is not whether this will be done, but only how, when, and to what extent.

Quality is in the eyes of the beholder, or customer. The secret of improving quality is focusing the attention of the whole organization on customers and instilling the concept that virtually everyone is both a supplier and a customer at different times.

Building a Culture of Continual Improvement

Hospitals and other healthcare organizations provide services and products to patients and their families. Many times, patients and families are under stress and feel very uncomfortable in an unfamiliar environment, yet many employees become casual, callous, and impersonal in their attitudes. What is equally bad is that employees may also treat one another poorly. Surveys can point out problems with interactions, whether they involve external or internal customers.

Whether we intend to or not, we create systems and incentives that reinforce our employees' acting the way they do. For example, we criticize employees for not working together to solve problems, yet we create performance plans and reward people for meeting individual goals. Team interaction is promoted with team goals, and each team member is evaluated for contributions to team goals. Rigid, decentralized departmental structures can inhibit people's working together.

Employees look to their leaders for clues about what is really important. One statement that conveys the need for congruent action is "Your actions speak so loudly that I cannot hear you." Unless leaders' actions are consistent with stated missions and values, progress toward transformation will be slowed or stopped. In subsequent chapters, we will address some actions, types of feedback, and types of incentives that enable congruent actions and words.

Promoting Innovation and Creativity

Successful organizations eliminate barriers to creativity. Any organization that can capture the innovative and creative abilities of its employees has a major advantage over its competitors. Employees who come to work every day, accomplish the tasks they are assigned, and leave without making creative contributions are often very creative in their outside lives. The secret is to stimulate, celebrate, and reward innovation and creativity, and tap into the potential of all employees.

Reorganizing the Way People Work and Interact

Most healthcare organizations have reorganized in the past decade, and many have had several top-down reorganizations, but few such reorganizations have significantly affected the way work is accomplished. In most cases, while organizational entities have been established, consolidated, or eliminated, these modifications have not changed the authority or responsibilities of employees, nor, in most cases, have they reduced the cross-departmental barriers that exist in healthcare organizations.

Reorganizing how work is accomplished means reviewing the actual performance of work—what gets done by whom—and the most effective methods.

Self-directed work groups, flattened hierarchy, and revised communication channels are all part of work reorganization and require new relationships among management and staff. Leaders must establish and demonstrate new behaviors and serve as role models and mentors during change processes. For example, nursing in the past decade moved in the direction of having an entire staff made up of baccalaureate-educated, professionally registered nurses; now, with the nurse shortage, new models to accomplish work are being explored.

Promoting Success as Everyone's Role

Closely related to cultural change is the concept that the organization's success is the responsibility of everyone who works there. Few employees give much thought to the possibility of their organization going out of business, particularly in large organizations, yet more and more healthcare organizations are going out of business or being acquired by larger corporations. Group and individual performance expectations should be directly tied to the success of the organization. An applicant should understand the basic corporate culture and values, as well as his or her role as an employee, before being hired. Supervisors should use interview time to assess whether a candidate will fit into the organizational culture and be a team player.

Improving Cost-Effectiveness

Most healthcare organizations have been undertaking cost-reduction programs. Many must cut costs to offset past or projected financial losses. Improving cost-effectiveness is an absolutely essential component of transformation; if undertaken inappropriately, however, cost cutting can destroy the human relationships necessary for accomplishing other components of transformation. Cost reduction is not always synonymous with improved cost-effectiveness; rash, unfeeling layoffs destroy an organization more than they position it for the future. Improved cost-effectiveness is a by-product of total quality, work reorganization, innovation, creativity, and management with quantitative information. The need for and value of the current organizational structure should be challenged. Reducing the size of an organization (downsizing) is one method of improving productivity and cost-effectiveness.

Managing with Quantitative and Qualitative Information

Information is crucial to informed management decisions, particularly in large organizations. Leaders must know how their organizations are performing and be able to simulate or evaluate alternatives before making decisions. It is becoming common practice for HMOs, PPOs, and other healthcare payers to seek competitive bids for services. To bid appropriately, healthcare decision makers must have accurate information on variable and total costs. Bid too high, and you lose business; bid too low, and you lose money on the business you get.

Leaders need timely access to many different measures of

internal performance, including information on work loads, staffing, productivity, quality, budget, costs, and utilization. Leaders also need timely information about current and potential customers, customers' perceptions and requirements, and competitors' measures of performance. The need for and use of quantitative information is, however, no substitute for judgment, decisions, and actions. Leaders and the organizations may benefit from multidisciplinary decision-support groups who analyze information and prepare it for managers.

Rethinking Strategies for Leadership Effectiveness

For your organization to be successful in the future, executives and managers at every level must become more effective leaders. Management development is an investment in people. Many organizations say, "People are our most important asset," and yet they provide few opportunities for education, training, or development.

Chapter Four

Revitalizing the Organization's Mission and Values

The first step of transformation is to prepare and present a compelling vision for the future as a guide to change. Transformation is painful, and employees will resist embarking on a major new journey unless they perceive that the change will be better than the current course.

The vision for the future will serve as the basis for reviewing and revitalizing your organization. The purpose of this chapter is to define the rationale, the likely outcomes, and the specific actions necessary to revitalization.

Without defined mission, values, and goals, it is folly to think that an organization can effectively achieve any collective goals. Every person will have his or her own perceptions of the purpose of the organization, and these will differ radically.

Leading a successful transformation requires both logical direction and emotional commitment. Therefore, the vision, mission, and values must have strong emotional appeal, in addition to a logical basis. Emotional appeal is important in creating the commitment and effort to undertake and endure the risks, problems, and hard work that are necessary to a successful implementation of major organizational change. The strategy is to begin by defining a vision or direction for the organization. This vision must be broadly communicated and consistent with personal values. We believe that successful leaders will use this vision to inspire and empower employees to create the world of work that they desire.

Definitions

Definitions vary from one organization to another. Consistency of definitions among organizations is nice but not

65

particularly important. Consistent, well-understood definitions within your organization, however, are critical. The following definitions are offered here to facilitate understanding of terms we use in this book.

Mission. This is the basic purpose of your organization. The mission statement often names types of products and services, customers, market areas, and other basic characteristics of the business. The mission statement should address the questions what, who, for whom, when, where, and why.

Vision. The guide to where your organization is going. This is particularly important if leaders see the need for a substantial change in direction.

Goals and Objectives. Goals are specific outcomes that you expect of your organization as a whole, or of specific segments of your organization. Objectives are stated in specific terms and have time frames assigned (for example, "meet affirmative action goals by next July").

Values. These are the basic beliefs that are most important to your organization and its workers.

Principles. These are the fundamental rules, doctrines, or assumptions by which you expect managers and other employees to act. Principles support values and establish basic priorities and fundamental expectations.

Statements of Mission and Values

Virtually every hospital and healthcare organization that we know of has a written mission statement. You probably have one as well, but what does it mean to you and your employees? Most mission statements try to be all things to all people at all times. They are so all-encompassing that they have no real meaning to most employees. Consider for a moment what employees see:

1. The mission, if written, may still not be effectively communicated. It is unlikely that every employee sees, much less has in his or her possession, a copy of the statements by which you direct your organization.
2. The written mission is likely to be so all-encompassing that it provides little direction.
3. Directions given by top, middle, and first-line managers are not consistent with the mission, and the discrepancies cause conflicts in directions and priorities.

What are employees supposed to do? Faced with many unprioritized and often conflicting directions, employees either withdraw into a very narrow view of their jobs or determine their own personal directions and priorities. For example, employees may say that their own units are fine and that they are pleased with work, but that other units are not so good. In this case, employees feel less commitment to the organization than to their units.

Action Step: **Read your written statements of mission and goals and answer the following questions.**

1. **Are the statements really clear?**
2. **Has every employee seen and received personal copies of these statements?**
3. **Do the statements address your mission and/ or vision, the basic values of your organization, and the principles by which managers and staff are expected to relate to one another?**
4. **Do everyday activities support the mission, or is there a gap between promise and performance?**

Action Step: **Ask a sample of employees to read the written statements of mission and goals. Ask those employees to state in their own words what**

**the statements mean to them. Do the employees
have a clear and consistent enough understanding to use the statements on their jobs?**

If you answer no to any of the preceding questions, your
statements will not allow effective communication of the organization's purpose to your staff, and the statements must be revised
and/or communicated.

The vision, as well as mission and values statements, must
address long-term questions: What business are we in? Why do
we exist? What human and business characteristics do we value?
What are the roles of research and education?

The mission statement must be couched in terms easily
understood by everyone — board members, employees, and customers. In addition, simple statements of the organization's
values and principles are important in guiding employees toward identification with the goals of the organization. More
important, these simple statements develop employees' sense of
how their roles fit with organizational goals.

We suggest that you also consider developing a statement
that captures the personal values of your employees and allows
them to see how their roles fit into the larger whole. Institutional
values should be consistent with personal values and should
arouse emotional commitment. One method of identifying employees' values and developing employees' buy-in is to organize
focus groups of employees and managers for discussion of organizational values and mission. Comments can then be synthe-
sized and developed into draft statements that employees can
understand. While these statements are being developed, there
should be broad involvement of employees. It will also be helpful to have others read these statements and to determine
whether they understand the message. Share drafts with employees and selected customers. Do not just ask people if they
understand the statements; ask them to tell you in their own
terms what the statements mean. Consistency of understanding
is key.

The values statements in Exhibits 1, 2, and 3 are from the
University of Michigan Medical Center in Ann Arbor, NKC

Exhibit 1. University of Michigan Medical Center Statement of Quality.

The University of Michigan Hospitals exist to meet the University's objectives in education, research and service. This mission is accomplished through people and knowledge, our most important resources. In the continuing pursuit of total quality, we are guided by the following values:

Respect: We will recognize the worth, quality, diversity and importance of each other, the people we serve, and the institution.

Compassion: We will care about others and respect their feelings.

Integrity: We will be honest and forthright and meet the highest ethical standards.

Efficiency: We will meet society's expectations and our own responsibility to be prudent with our resources.

Excellence: We will work together to be the very best in everything we do.

Source: University of Michigan Medical Center. Reprinted with permission.

Hospitals, Inc., in Louisville, Kentucky, and Ford Motor Company in Dearborn, Michigan. All three organizations distribute laminated cards containing their statements to all employees. The University of Michigan Medical Center established its values with focus groups of employees, physicians, managers, and executives. Trained facilitators asked group members about the values that they felt their organization should espouse in the 1990s and beyond. Results of the group sessions were collated and shown to the chief executive officer, the chief operating officer, and the director of planning and marketing, who drafted statements of values on the basis of this information and their own visions for the future. The draft statements were then redistributed for comments and editing. Statements of mission and values convey to every employee, customer, and supplier, in simple terms, the values of the organization and the ethical and interpersonal behaviors that are desired.

In 1987, the Maryland Hospital Association called for its member hospitals to develop corporate ethics, which, along with biomedical ethics, would be the cornerstones of their credibility in their communities. According to a report to the board (Maryland Hospital Association, 1987), these ethics will be the

Exhibit 2. NKC Corporate Values and Quality Policy.

Corporate Values

Respect for every individual
Delivery of quality service
Constant pursuit of excellence

NKC Quality Policy

Quality in everything we do and every decision we make is an attitude which we must create and nurture. We will provide those served, externally and internally, with services which conform to clearly established requirements.

We will design or modify the ways we do our work in order to constantly make improvements and to prevent errors. This will assure that the right things are done the right way each and every time.

It is management's role to support employees by eliminating barriers to efficiency and quality. All employees and each supplier to NKC must adopt our standards of quality in accordance with our mission, goals and values.

Source: NKC Hospitals. Reprinted with permission.

answer to two key questions: Are they doing the right things? Are they doing them well? The report goes on to state that as hospitals adjust to changes in their environments and respond to calls for greater cost containment, higher-quality care, and more businesslike behavior, they will face many tests of their ability to make business and policy decisions that are true to their mission and values, sensitive and fair to their employees, and in the best interests of the patients and the communities they serve. The report supports the view that a hospital's values and ethics should permeate its planning, marketing, restructuring, and joint venturing, as well as its delivery of services, quality assessment, employee relations, and financial management. The report also defines *corporate ethics* as the organization's values and standards expressed in action through the organization's roles as caregiver, employer, buyer, seller, business partner, and member of the community it serves.

Well-defined mission, values, and principles are the basis of all the other components of transformation. As a secondary benefit of defining these elements in terms that all employees can understand and support, specific policies and procedures become less important. When the message is unclear, however,

Exhibit 3. Ford Motor Company's Mission, Values, and Guiding Principles.

Mission: Ford Motor Company is a worldwide leader in automotive and automotive-related products and services, as well as in newer industries, such as aerospace, communications, and financial services. Our mission is to improve continually our products and services to meet our customers' needs, allowing us to prosper as a business and to provide a reasonable return for our stockholders, the owners of the business.

Values: How we accomplish our mission is as important as the mission itself. Fundamental to success for the Company are these basic values:

People: Our people are the source of our strength. They provide our corporate intelligence and determine our reputation and vitality. Involvement and teamwork are our core human values.

Products: Our products are the end result of our efforts, and they should be the best in serving customers worldwide. As our products are viewed, so are we viewed.

Profits: Profits are the ultimate measure of how efficiently we provide customers with the best products for their needs. Profits are required to survive and grow.

Guiding Principles

Quality comes first. To achieve customer satisfaction, the quality of our products and services must be our number one priority.

Customers are the focus of everything we do. Our work must be done with our customers in mind, providing better products and services than our competition.

Employee involvement is our way of life. We must strive for excellence in everything we do in our products, in their safety and value — and in our services, our human relations, our competitiveness, and our profitability.

Continuous improvement is essential to our success. We are a team. We must treat each other with trust and respect.

Dealers and suppliers are our partners. The Company must maintain mutually beneficial relationships with dealers, suppliers, and our other business associates.

Integrity is never compromised. The conduct of our Company worldwide must be pursued in a manner that is socially responsible and commands respect for its integrity and for its positive contributions to society. Our doors are open to men and women alike without discrimination and without regard to ethnic origin or personal beliefs.

Source: Ford Motor Company. Reprinted with permission.

management must respond to each of many potential circumstances with a unique policy or procedure. As we have said, such specific policies and procedures consume substantial resources and tend to limit creativity.

Recognizing Multiple Goals

Establishing clear statements of purpose is not simple in healthcare organizations. Virtually no organization has a single goal; but healthcare organizations have multiple, often conflicting, goals. Americans believe that healthcare organizations are special social institutions; thus, development of clear standards will help us reestablish ourselves in our communities.

Taxonomy of Healthcare Services

One useful approach to understanding and evaluating alternative roles for your organization is to formally consider a cross-classification, or *taxonomy*, of healthcare services. One taxonomy of healthcare services was developed by Richard J. Coffey at Chi Systems, Inc., for the Canadian government (Canadian Department of National Health and Welfare, 1979). This taxonomy organizes all health and medical services into four dimensions, described in the paragraphs that follow.

Patient's Condition. This is a classification of the patient's medical or health condition. One type of classification of ill patients employs diagnosis-related groups, or DRGs, which are used by the U.S. Department of Health and Human Services to reimburse for care provided to Medicare patients. Clearly, a classification of well people supplements any classification of ill patients. The patient's condition is the basis for many of the product lines currently being developed and marketed by healthcare organizations.

Functions. These are groups of different activities, organized by type of focus. One way to divide functions is according to promotion, protection, prevention, detection, diagnosis, treatment, habilitation and rehabilitation, maintenance, support, education, research, and enabling.

Settings. These are the physical locations where medical and healthcare services are provided. A setting may be a whole area (especially in areawide health-promotion campaigns using television, radio, or billboards), or it may be the home, work, or school, as well as social, mobile, ambulatory, inpatient, and freestanding support sites.

Resources. This category includes people, buildings and equipment, money, organizations, and information.

The taxonomy could be used in a hospital, for example, in developing a new hypertension-control program. The focus of the program would be the *condition* of hypertension, or high blood pressure. *Functions* to be included in the program might be health promotion, prevention, and detection, and patients could be referred to the medical staff for diagnosis, treatment, and rehabilitation. Since people with hypertension are sometimes unaware of their condition, the most appropriate *settings* for promotion, prevention, and detection might be work and ambulatory-care environments. Appropriate *resources* might include nurse clinicians who would use mobile testing equipment, which could be set up in shopping centers and places of employment.

In addition to using taxonomies of healthcare services, many healthcare organizations are initiating a wide variety of for-profit ventures outside healthcare. Examples of non-healthcare ventures include real-estate investment and management, hotels, restaurants, landscaping, and transportation. It is very important to determine the purposes of such external ventures in relation to the overall mission, values, and principles of the organization.

> *Action Step*: **With your board, physicians, customers, and managers, review the taxonomy of healthcare services, nonhealthcare ventures, and appropriate roles for your organization. Establish priorities and interrelationships with your board so that the plan will be achievable.**

Clinical Care, Education, and Research

Apart from its many different services, described in the taxonomy, the basic purpose of the organization must be established. In such community healthcare organizations as hospitals, nursing homes, and home-care agencies, the clear purpose is normally to provide healthcare services and products in the most cost-effective manner. In academic health centers, however, purposes are less clear. The purpose of a university is to develop and disseminate new knowledge through research, development, publication, and education. The priorities vary among clinical care, education, and research. For an academic health center, then, it is particularly important that mission, values, and goals be clear, so that employees understand them. For example, a clinic manager may face somewhat conflicting objectives. Faculty may place importance on academic exposure for students and time for research; patients want timely and considerate service from experienced physicians. Such circumstances are common in teaching hospitals and academic health centers. In the absence of clear and communicated mission, values, and goals, every physician, manager, and patient will act only as he or she feels is appropriate.

Priorities of Goals

Much more difficult than defining the different goals of your organization will be determining their priorities, particularly the priorities of conflicting goals. Involvement of customers, managers, and employees is important for informed decisions about priorities.

Involvement to Develop Mission and Values

While establishing mission, values, and principles is the responsibility of the organization's leaders, that does not mean that leaders create these in a vacuum, without input from others. Input and discussion during development are crucial to achieving support from the people involved. Specific input should be sought from the groups described in this section.

Leaders in Your Organization. You should conduct a formal survey of the opinions of your board and senior managers for two reasons. First, you can determine individual opinions without the bias of the group's peer pressure. This will reveal the initial consistency or inconsistency of perceived values. Second, you gain statistical information about group opinion and deviations from what will become the corporate mission and values. Once mission, values, principles, and goals are established, however, leaders in your organization must actively and consistently support them. Those who cannot must leave.

Customers. Customers include patients, other healthcare consumers, and many more groups. At least four customer groups should be involved in revitalizing your values:

1. *Patients.* Although they have often been overlooked, patients' viewpoints are very important in establishing the goals of an organization. The days when experts decided what was good for the customer are over. As reimbursement for services becomes even more restricted, we must understand the views of patients and physicians, in order to set priorities for our services.
2. *Physicians.* Although physicians are always considered key customers of healthcare organizations, few organizations formally involve them at all levels in developing statements of mission, values, and principles. In some cases, physicians may also be employees.
3. *Employees.* Employees are unique in that they are important internal customers as well as providers of the services offered by your organization. Nevertheless, how often have you formally solicited input from your employees to establish or revise your mission, values, and principles? There are two useful approaches. First, you can convene focus groups of employees, to determine their perceptions of appropriate statements of mission, vision, values, principles, and so on. A random sample of representative employees is most valid because it is likely to represent the complete range of opinion. Using "employees of the month" or volunteers is also helpful but may involve a bias toward current actions. Second, you can distribute a survey questionnaire to em-

ployees (to all or to a sample). The wording of questions should minimize bias and be simple enough for all employ- ees to understand. It may be helpful to have focus groups identify issues and then develop a survey questionnaire, to gain a broader representation of opinions. It is useful to think of the people whom patients and their family mem- bers see every day: physicians, nurses, dietetics staff, house- keeping staff, receptionists, aides, door and parking lot attendants, and other first-line employees. These are the people who must convey your corporate image.

4.   *Payers.* Business, industry, government, and union leaders are also customers and will be exerting more pressure for change. Asking payers for feedback can provide valuable insights. One of the world's largest healthcare providers, Hospital Corporation of America, has developed formal survey questionnaires that are regularly administered to patients, physicians, payers, and employees. These differ from typical patient surveys in that they document both positive and negative perceptions and are used to change the services provided to customers (Spechler, 1988).

Suppliers. Organizations and people providing services and products to your organization may also be able to help you develop your mission and values. More important, their involve- ment will make your mission and values clear to them, so that they can better meet your requirements.

Related Organizations. Input from superior, subordinate, and related organizations is necessary in establishing mission and values, particularly when a healthcare organization is part of a university, a government agency, or a multihospital chain. In these cases, the goals of the university or agency may set limits or priorities on your mission and values.

> *Action Step*: **Obtain formal and informal input from customers, leaders, employees, and sup- pliers about your mission, values, and principles. Regular input from these same groups is a key**

to continual improvement of quality and performance.

After input has been obtained from these sources, it is the leaders' responsibility to synthesize that information and develop the statements of mission, values, and principles. Leaders must exercise breadth of vision for the future and integrate priorities among competing goals and segments of the organization. We suggest a day-long retreat with board members, key physician leaders, and the senior management team to review information from focus groups and other sources and to develop the statements.

Action Step: **Integrate the information and perceptions of others to develop clear statements of the mission, values, and principles of your organization.**

Hierarchy of Goals

As you work to establish your corporate mission, values, goals, and principles, it is important to visualize how these will be translated into the goals of individual divisions, departments, entities, and people. The basic values and guiding principles should remain constant throughout your organization. For example, if your organization values people as its primary resource, then this value should be reflected throughout the organization.

The organization's goals should be reasonably specific about the types of specialized services that will be provided. Given the strong competition, it is increasingly difficult to be all things to all people. Focusing goals on specific customers' requirements will help focus employees' actions; this approach is known as *market segmentation*.

There is, however, a hierarchy of missions and goals, as illustrated in Figure 6. The mission of each department should be stated in the context of the corporate mission, but with specifics related to that department. Another way of visualizing

Figure 6. Hierarchy of Mission and Goals.

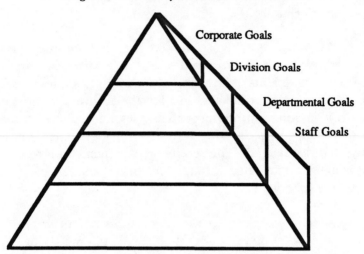

the relationship of goals is illustrated in Figure 7. Departmental goals will be more detailed than organizational goals. For example, the mission of the radiology department may be to provide a variety of imaging services at several locations while fulfilling the hospital's general mission. Ultimately, each employee should be able to see how his or her performance goals are related to the mission and goals of the organization.

Communication of Mission, Values, and Principles

A mission, a vision, goals, values, and principles are of little consequence unless all employees know, understand, and implement them. The following methods are useful in communicating mission and values to employees:

1. State the organizational values in all employment literature. Discuss the values during interviews, to hire candidates who share them.
2. Include specific discussion of mission, values, and principles in every new employee's orientation.

Figure 7. Relationship of Goals.

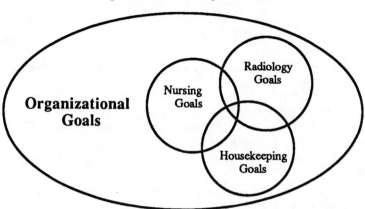

3. Pass out copies of mission and value statements to every employee.

4. Ask employees to restate the mission and values in their own words, frequently. You could offer tokens of recognition and incentives to employees who know the mission and values; honor them in your organizational newsletter, for example.

5. Make management's decisions and actions consistent with the stated mission and values. This is most important, since people will believe what they see in action. Michael Bice, former chief executive officer of Lutheran Health System, calls management personnel who behave consistently with stated values executives who "walk their talk."

> *Action Step*: **Distribute a copy of your mission and values statement to every employee, preferably on a small card that is easily carried.**

Management Expectations

The next step in transformation is to develop management expectations. In our experience, healthcare organizations are not explicit about what they expect from managers and

Exhibit 4. University of Michigan Medical Center's Management Expectations.

Each of us will act in accordance with the overall purpose of the University of Michigan Medical Center.

Each of us will create and support an environment which fosters teamwork, emphasizes quality, and promotes learning.

Each of us will create and support an environment that builds on the contribution of every employee.

Each of us will promote cooperation and coordination among individuals and departments to provide the best system of care and customer service.

We will live the Quality Process by constantly making improvements, preventing errors, and continually striving to:

I. Develop and support a work environment where every employee's capability is improved.

Recognize that every employee wants to be a valued contributor and is capable of making an important contribution.

Select and promote based on individual strengths, knowledge, leadership skills and ability to work as part of a team.

Provide a complete orientation to employees of their work areas.

Insure that employees understand what is needed from them.

Provide employees with thorough on-going training to do their jobs.

Give continual feedback regarding assessment of their job performance.
  Identify and compliment individuals on the areas in which they are performing well.
  Problem solve with employees to help employees improve their work.

Identify and remove barriers that prevent employees from improvement.

Challenge employees to improve by providing the environment, training and skills needed.

Identify employee strengths and place employees in positions where they can make the greatest contributions.

Identify, with employees, opportunities for their development.

II. Develop an environment where individuals are an integral part of the improvement process.

Recognize that employees possess the expertise to make decisions about their jobs.

Share and give authority to individuals to resolve problems.

Solicit employee input and utilize that input.

Follow up on previously identified opportunities for improvement.

Involve and cooperate with other departments in pursuing opportunities for improvement.

Involve employees in interdepartmental problem solving.

Encourage an action orientation.

**Exhibit 4. University of Michigan Medical Center's
Management Expectations, Cont'd.**

III. Promote an environment of open communication.

Share information with employees to give them a macro view about:
Healthcare trends
Organizational trends
Financial data
Departmental goals, achievements, and overall performance
Provide information to employees which allows them to perform their job[s].
Interact with employees on a regular basis.
Be clear when delegating regarding:
The goals, objectives of the assignment
Performance measures
Expectations regarding communication
The amount of authority they have to complete the assignment
Conduct meetings for information sharing and problem solving on a regular basis.
Share appreciation of employees' contributions.
Utilize effective listening skills by not interrupting, not assuming you know what is being said, by asking clarifying questions and letting [employees] know your understanding of what they said.
In speaking and working with employees, enhance or maintain their self-esteem.
Solicit input from employees.

IV. Create an atmosphere that promotes and encourages innovation and creativity.

Accept mistakes as a normal part of trying something new.
Respond to mistakes with constructive criticism; learn from them.
Consider errors as opportunities for improvement.
Demonstrate willingness to cooperate with others.
Encourage and sponsor quality improvement ideas.
Reward employees for participation and innovation through recognition, appreciation and celebration.

V. Foster an environment which values diversity and sustains multiculturalism.

Examine your own cultural background to understand how your frame of reference can lead to misunderstanding and miscommunication with others.
Learn more about the culture of diverse groups in order to understand and respect their cultural values, customs and viewpoint[s].
Select and develop employees based on their strengths. Learn how to avoid stereotyping and avoid the tendency to pass value judgments on others.
Promote respect and build on the differences of those in the work group.

Source: University of Michigan Medical Center, "Expectations of Management." Reprinted with permission.

supervisors. Organizations often promote excellent clinicians to management roles, without giving them formal management education or informal mentoring. Somehow, the new managers are expected to absorb what they need through osmosis.

We suggest forming a task force of representative managers to develop a set of expectations that flow from the mission and values. Management expectations should be clearly defined in behavioral terms. Exhibit 4 reproduces the University of Michigan Medical Center's management expectations.

> *Action Step*: **Distribute copies of the management expectations to every supervisor and manager. Review the expectations with candidates before hiring any new manager or supervisor. Use the expectations to evaluate managers, and reward behaviors in a way that is consistent with the stated expectations.**

Mission, values, and management expectations all establish the basic beliefs and expectations for board members, employees, physicians, customers, and suppliers. These should be widely distributed and posted in prominent locations. They should serve as the framework for all decisions and actions.

Chapter Five

❧❧❧❧

Establishing
a Total Quality Process

Quality is clearly one of the most talked about, most important, and most pursued topics of this decade. Many corporations in the United States are in some stage of consideration or implementation of a total quality approach. Quality is important as a focus for improving services and products, as a marketing strategy, and as a method of improving cost-effectiveness.

Quality became popularized when several American industries (electronics, automobiles, and cameras) lost market share to Japan. These corporations found themselves in a grave situation. Once known as producers of shoddy goods, the Japanese had made quality a goal, and they began to produce goods perceived to be of superior quality. Simply stated, the quality of American products had to improve, or many major corporations would continue to lose market share and possibly go bankrupt. Americans and other consumers worldwide were and are demanding higher-quality products and services at competitive prices.

Many hospitals and healthcare organizations find themselves in a similar situation today. They are experiencing strong competition in an industry with excess capacity. A new emphasis on quality can refocus and reposition healthcare organizations to compete more effectively.

A number of experts in the United States offer assistance in developing quality programs with industrial methods. Probably the three best-known experts are W. Edwards Deming, Joseph Juran, and Philip Crosby. Each advocates a somewhat different approach to quality improvement, but the underlying principles are the same.

83

Definitions of Customers and Quality

One problem associated with quality is knowing how to define it. Quality is a difficult concept to define because it exists essentially in the eyes of the beholder. Each person defines quality somewhat differently, and the definition may change over time.

The concept of quality medical care is complex and does not have a single, generally accepted definition. According to Donabedian (1980, p. 27), "there are several definitions of quality, or several variants of a single definition; and . . . each definition or variant is legitimate in its appropriate context." Donabedian and other authorities have measured quality through the attributes of structure, process, and outcome, and this is the approach used by most healthcare quality-assurance committees. Hospitals have had such committees for decades, but these bodies have focused narrowly on components of clinical care, such as reviews of tissues removed during surgery, types of tests, medications, and procedures for patients with certain diagnoses, and selected medical outcomes. Whether they have been focusing on structure, process, or outcome, quality has been defined internally by the healthcare professions and accrediting bodies. The approaches used by quality-assurance committees are important and useful but can be even stronger when combined with some of the broader quality-improvement techniques used in other industries.

In healthcare, many people have legitimate roles in defining and evaluating quality—patients, physicians, nurses, patients' families and friends, co-workers, leaders and managers, professional associations, third-party payers, employers, and others. Clearly, criteria for measuring quality, as well as the relative importance of quality itself, may vary widely among these individuals.

It is important to define the terms *customer* and *supplier*, as well as their relationship to each other and to quality. *Customer* is an all-inclusive term that is much broader than *patient*; it includes patients' families, physicians, nurses, other healthcare professionals, co-workers, professional associations, and third-

Figure 8. Supplier-Customer Relationship.

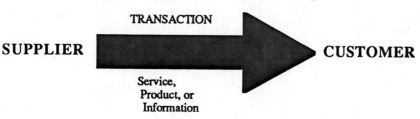

TRANSACTION

SUPPLIER   CUSTOMER

Service,
Product, or
Information

party payers. A simple way of visualizing the supplier-customer relationship is illustrated in Figure 8. For any transaction involving a product, service, or information, the person or organization at the tail of the arrow is the supplier, and the person or organization at the head of the arrow is the customer. For any transaction in which you are providing something to someone else, that person is the customer.

Internal as well as external customers are involved. Internal customers are normally those within your organization, and external customers are those outside. The reason for this distinction is the degree to which you can influence and negotiate customers' requirements. With external customers, you may have no ability to negotiate requirements. A referring physician, for example, may require that referred patients be seen within forty-eight hours of referral. If you fail to meet this requirement, the physician may refer patients elsewhere. With internal customers, you are usually able to negotiate requirements if you feel that they are unrealistic.

Supplier-customer roles switch for different transactions; every person is both a supplier and a customer at different times. The key is to understand the requirements of each transaction, so that the supplier can meet them.

Figure 9 illustrates the changing customer-supplier relationships for the process of providing medications. At each step in this process, the customer and the supplier change, and each person depends on the accuracy and timeliness of the information that he or she receives to perform his or her job correctly. If

Figure 9. Customer-Supplier Relationships for Medication Order.

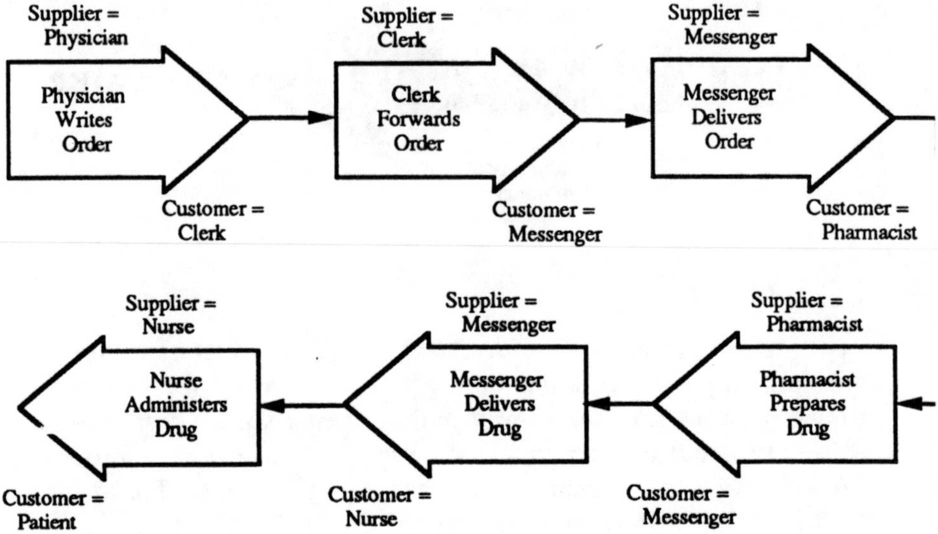

Supplier =
Physician

Physician
Writes
Order

Customer =
Clerk

Supplier =
Clerk

Clerk
Forwards
Order

Customer =
Messenger

Supplier =
Messenger

Messenger
Delivers
Order

Customer =
Pharmacist

Supplier =
Nurse

Nurse
Administers
Drug

Customer =
Patient

Supplier =
Messenger

Messenger
Delivers
Drug

Customer =
Nurse

Supplier =
Pharmacist

Pharmacist
Prepares
Drug

Customer =
Messenger

the physician does not write legibly or orders medication that is not in the formulary, then the pharmacist cannot fill the order. Therefore, the messenger cannot deliver it to the nurse, who in turn cannot administer it to the patient.

We believe that quality must be defined in terms of some expected use or outcome, as judged by the customer. There is always a judgment involved. For example, a waiting time of thirty minutes could be judged acceptable and relatively short by the physicians in a clinic, but it could also be judged unacceptable by patients in the same clinic.

Quality, then, can be defined in a number of ways. For Juran (1988), product performance means satisfaction and freedom from deficiencies. For Crosby (1979, p. 15), quality is "conformance to requirements." According to Ishikawa (1985, p. 44), "The Japanese Industrial Standards...define quality control as follows: 'A system of production methods which economically produces quality goods or services meeting the requirements of consumers. Modern quality control utilizes statistical methods and is often called statistical quality control.'" And for Deming (1986, pp. 168–169), "Quality can be defined only in terms of the agent. Who is the judge of quality? In the mind of the production worker, he produces quality if he can take pride in his work. . . . The quality of any product or service has many scales. A product may get a high mark, in the judgment of the consumer, on one scale, and a low mark on another."

Contrast the following interpretations of quality. A person wanting basic transportation might consider a Toyota or Ford Escort to be a quality automobile. A person wanting a luxurious ride, a fine interior, many additional features, and the status related to the car's limited production might consider a Rolls-Royce to be a quality automobile. The concept of quality is closely linked to the concept of value for the price paid.

An example from the healthcare industry is the type of room one requires. Historically, a bed in a ward with a community shower and toilet met the customer's requirements and was considered acceptable. Today, customers' requirements include a private or semiprivate room, a private bathroom, a telephone, and a television. There is no absolute measure of quality; it depends on the requirements of the customer. Given the wide variety of customers, expectations, and conditions, the simplest and easiest way to define *quality* is to say that it refers to whatever meets customers' requirements.

QUALITY = MEETING VALID REQUIREMENTS OF THE CUSTOMER

Inherent in most customers' requirements is an expectation of both service and value. Historically, most organizations have excluded external and some internal customer representatives from formal processes that were intended to define and evaluate quality. Nevertheless, customers should be directly involved in defining both their own requirements and the measures of quality. Likewise, every organization must determine its own definition of quality and processes to improve quality and must communicate these throughout the organization.

Action Step: **Define *quality* as the term that will be used in your organization and communicate that definition to everyone.**

Figure 10. The Juran Trilogy.

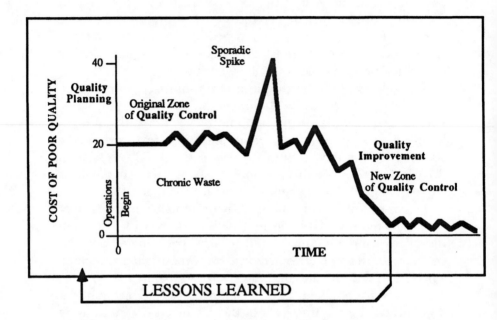

Source: Juran, 1987. Reproduced with the permission of the Juran Institute.

Complementing definitions of quality are processes to manage and improve quality. Juran (1987) has developed a useful schema for viewing three different processes relating to quality (the schema is known as the Juran Trilogy):

1. *Quality planning* is the process of planning and designing processes to produce high quality. At this stage, the greatest gains can be made in designing processes, products, and services to avoid quality problems. Quality planning precedes the measurements graphed in Figure 10.
2. *Quality control* is the process of monitoring quality and managing it within the control limits achievable through

the current process. The left part of the graph in Figure 10 illustrates the original quality-control zone for the process, and the right part of the graph illustrates the new zone of quality control after quality improvement.

3. *Quality improvement* involves improving current processes. This goal is normally accomplished with a series of projects to improve quality. The most effective projects cross traditional departmental or corporate lines. The section of the graph in Figure 10 showing the steady, sharp decline reflects the results of quality-improvement efforts.

Juran's three processes have their analogies with familiar financial processes. Quality planning corresponds to budgeting, quality control to cost control, and quality improvement to cost reduction and margin improvement.

Quality may exist in fact and in perception. Most kinds of services, products, and information can be evaluated in terms of both fact and perception. Quality in fact is normally judged by professionals, with quantitative measures. An example of such judgment would be the measures established by the Joint Commission on Accreditation of Healthcare Organizations (JCAHO). Other examples might involve judgments about service times, waiting times, and the temperature of food. Quality in perception is a subjective evaluation, particularly as judged by customers: "I will know quality when I see it." For example, a customer perceives that he was treated rudely, or that his questions were not answered. Perceptions about one service are often extrapolated to the other products and services of an organization, fairly or not. For example, if you find a filthy restroom in a restaurant, you may conclude that the kitchen is also dirty or that the food is of poor quality. Similarly, patients and other customers often judge the quality of one service or product according to their perceptions of other services. Customers will act in accordance with their perceptions, independent of quantitative measurements.

Quality and Process Improvement

Continual improvement in quality and processes has two important components. The first is a philosophy and attitude of seeking to continually improve quality for your customers. The second is the set of techniques and theories used to make improvements. In almost all cases, process improvements lead to improvements in quality and cost-effectiveness.

Philosophies and Attitudes of Quality Improvement

Certain philosophies and attitudes underlie almost all process improvements. These philosophies and attitudes must exist before improvement techniques can be helpful. Some of the most important philosophies, attitudes, and techniques are briefly summarized here.

Constancy of Purpose. The attitude that everyone in the organization should know the overall mission and goals is very important (see also Chapter Ten).

Customer Orientation. The focus on customers and their requirements is a key attitude for any organization seeking to provide the best quality of care; quality is defined by your customers.

Continual Improvement. An attitude of continually striving to improve is absolutely necessary to the total quality process improvement. If individuals or organizations consider their current performance adequate for the future, they will not look for ways to improve.

Benchmarking. One technique used by the best organizations in the world is benchmarking. In its classic form, this is the technique of searching worldwide for the very best example of each component of a product or service and then setting that standard as the minimum target for improvement (Garvin, 1988). (This standard is sometimes called "best in class" for each of the characteristics.) It is common for healthcare organizations to look for benchmarks in other local organizations or in those that offer the same range of services. However, for specialized services, national and even international benchmarking is appropriate.

People Who Perform Jobs Know Those Jobs Best. In seeking improvements, an important attitude is that people who perform jobs know those jobs best. Front-line employees must be an integral part of any quality-improvement team. Managers may understand jobs overall, but they are less familiar with the day-to-day details than the people who do those jobs every day.

Teamwork. While the performance of some individuals is noteworthy, the organization will succeed or fail on the team participation and effort of everyone.

Quality Is Built In. It is important for everyone to recognize that quality needs to be built into every process and product. The best you can do with quality-by-inspection is to prevent poor-quality items from reaching the customer. The inspection approach results in waste and rework, and poor-quality items still exist. The goal is to improve the process through prevention of defects and planning for quality.

Techniques of Quality Improvement

A whole series of techniques are useful for process improvement, but none will be very effective unless your managers, physicians, nurses, and other employees and suppliers are committed to customers and to meeting their requirements. A handy, pocket-size reference to tools and techniques is the *Memory Jogger* (GOAL/QPC, 1988). These tools and techniques are helpful in documenting, measuring, and evaluating opportunities and improvements:

1. *Brainstorming,* a structured or unstructured approach to generating many ideas. The ideas should not be challenged or evaluated during brainstorming; evaluation at an early stage limits creativity. (Example: a quality-improvement team working to reduce waiting time.)

2. *Nominal group technique*, a method of having a group set priorities and select opportunities for improvement. This technique avoids the disproportionate influence of forceful members. Surveys can be used, so that people never actually need to meet.

3. *Interviews and survey questionnaires*, approaches to gathering opinions.

4. *Flow charts*, pictorial representations of sequences of steps. A flow chart may represent physical movement, movement of information, or other characteristics. (See Figure 11.)

5. *Cause-effect, or fishbone, diagrams*, pictorial representations of all the possible causes of specified effects. Causes are outlined along four to five major branches, causing the final chart to look like a fishbone. (See Figure 12.)

6. *Checksheets*, simple forms to record, or check, the frequency of different events or opinions.

7. *Pie/bar graphs*, showing frequency or percentage data displayed as slices of a circle (or as bars) for different events.

8. *Histograms*, bar graphs of the frequency of different events or measurements; a checksheet can provide frequency data. (See Figure 13.)

9. *Pareto charts*, specialized histograms, or bar graphs, displaying the frequency of different problems in decreasing frequency. A Pareto chart is used to set priorities on opportunities for improvement. (See Figure 14.)

10. *Force-field analysis*, a tabular, side-by-side display of the driving and restraining forces for a potential change. "If the restraining forces are stronger than the driving forces, then the desired change does not happen" (GOAL/QPC, 1988, p. 73).

11. *Run charts*, line graphs of measurements over time (see Figure 15). The line graph on the chart in Figure 10 is another illustration of a run chart.

12. *Control charts*, run charts with the addition of upper and lower control limits. These limits are used to make judgments about when a process is out of control.

13. *Stratification*, a technique that divides a single set of numbers into two or more meaningful categories, or classifica-

Figure 11. Flow Chart of Elective Surgery Scheduling Process.

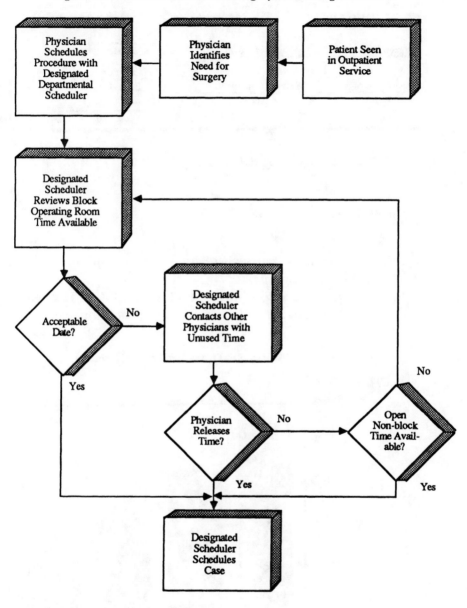

Figure 12. Fishbone Diagram of Reasons for Surgery Delays.

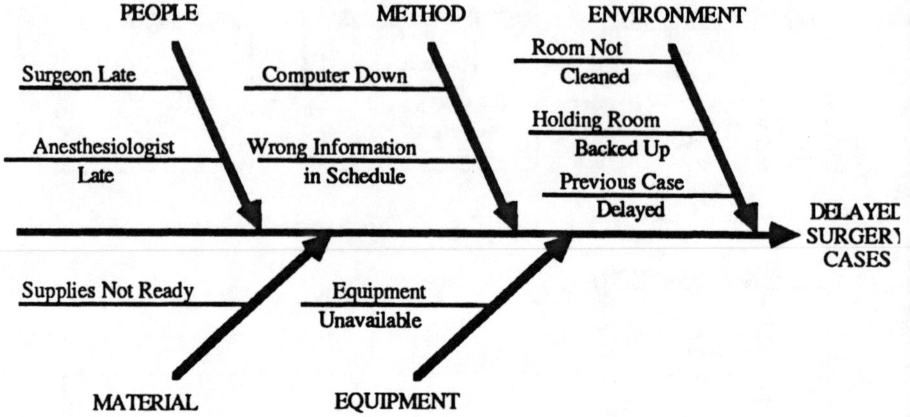

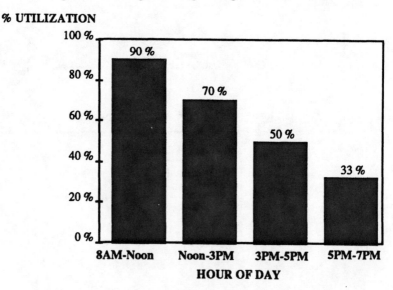

tions, to focus corrective action. This technique is also called *disaggregation*.

14. *Stability assessment*, a judgment of whether there has been any change in the underlying process generating measure-

Figure 13. Histogram of Operating Room Utilization.

Figure 14. Pareto Chart of Surgery Delays.

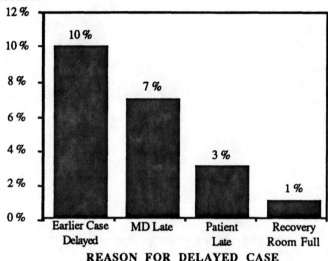

ments. The assessment is based on observations from a control chart of the measurements (Deming, 1986).

15. *Quality-function deployment*, a method of relating customers' demands, quality characteristics, and the quality plan (King, 1989).

Process Versus Departmental Focus

One of the keys to improvement is focusing on the process, rather than on the organizational unit, such as a clinical, nursing, ancillary, support, or administrative department in a healthcare organization. A *process* is the sequence of activities and communications that accomplish a service for a patient or other customer (for example, the admission/discharge process). Virtually every department has some function in the admission/discharge process; radiology performs admission X rays, nursing prepares a patient to leave, pharmacy prepares discharge medications, patient transportation escorts the patient, and so on. The traditional approach has been to focus budgeting and

Figure 15. Sample Run Chart of Waiting Times in Admitting.

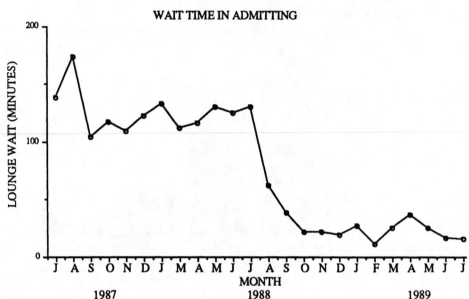

changes on the organizational units, as illustrated in Figure 16. With the focus on departments, processes receive a lower priority. Therefore, communications break down at departmental borders, and delays and other poor service result.

The recommended approach is to focus on the process, with less emphasis given to departments, as illustrated in Figure 17. Priority is given to organizational goals and customers, with lower priority given to departments. Some organizations have reorganized around product lines, to focus more on the processes associated with them, but departments continue to serve an important role in training and managing people with similar education and skills.

Theories for Process Improvement

Theories, as the term is used here, are ideas or hypotheses about how to improve a process, in terms of quality or some other measure of performance. Debate over whether a theory is

Figure 16. Departmental Focus.

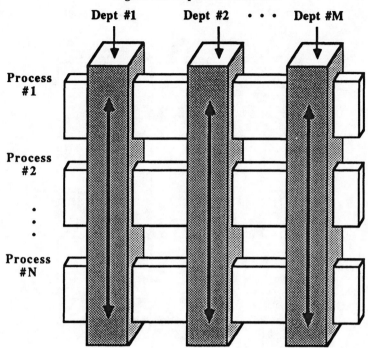

good or bad is generally unproductive; it is better simply to evaluate whether a theory is useful in improving performance of current processes (Rothman, 1989). While many theories have been offered to explain variations in processes, some theories have been found generally useful in improving most processes. In addition, the following factors are important:

1. *Consistent operational definitions*: Process variation is always reduced when consistent operational definitions are used.
2. *Single supplier*: Variation is always reduced with a smaller number of suppliers. A single, good supplier produces the least variation.
3. *Looking upstream*: The farther upstream a process can be improved, the better.
4. *Looking for rate-limiting steps*: Improving any steps that now

Figure 17. Process Focus.

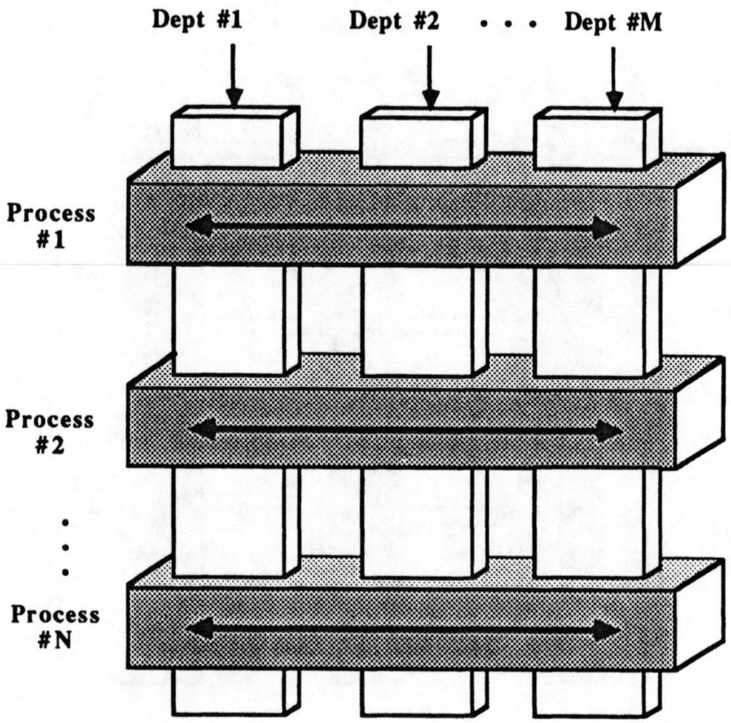

limit the rate or quality of output will yield the greatest results.

5. *Disaggregation:* Separating, or disaggregating, the sources of a service, product, or information will allow you to identify causes of variation more easily and improve processes. (Attention to this factor is similar to the use of a single supplier.)

Components of the Total Quality Process

The total quality process must be tailored to each organization, to make sure that it fits and will work in the existing culture. Different quality experts propose different approaches, and each has been successful. As we said earlier, however, the basic concepts are common to Deming, Juran, Crosby, and others.

Planning and Directing the Quality Process

Planning for quality is similar to planning for new programs and services, budgets, or any other major organizational activity. Quality is not a "quick fix" or just another program; it takes from five to ten years to fully implement a quality process. Quality needs to be thought of as a way of life. One approach that has been successful in several healthcare and industrial organizations will be briefly described here.

A quality council, or steering committee, should be established, to provide overall direction and make policy decisions related to the quality-improvement process. Participation should be broadly representative, with delegates from the medical staff, nursing, major ancillary departments, administration, and employee groups. To the extent possible, people with broad organizational vision and commitment should be appointed to the quality council, since the council will be planning the quality-improvement process to benefit the entire organization, including its patients and other customers.

A very important task of the quality council is the development of a plan, or roadmap, to change the organizational environment and culture. An example of such a plan is shown in Exhibit 5.

As specific policy or organizationwide issues arise, it is helpful to appoint task forces to address those issues. The role of a task force is to investigate the issue, develop alternatives, research the advantages and disadvantages of each, and recommend an action plan to the quality council. The council may request additional information, surveys, or action from the task force. After the council has made its policy decision and approved an action plan, the task force is dissolved. For example, the University of Michigan Hospitals established task forces to address vision and values, management commitment, work reorganization, rewards and recognition, communication and

Exhibit 5. University of Michigan Medical Center's Total Quality Roadmap.

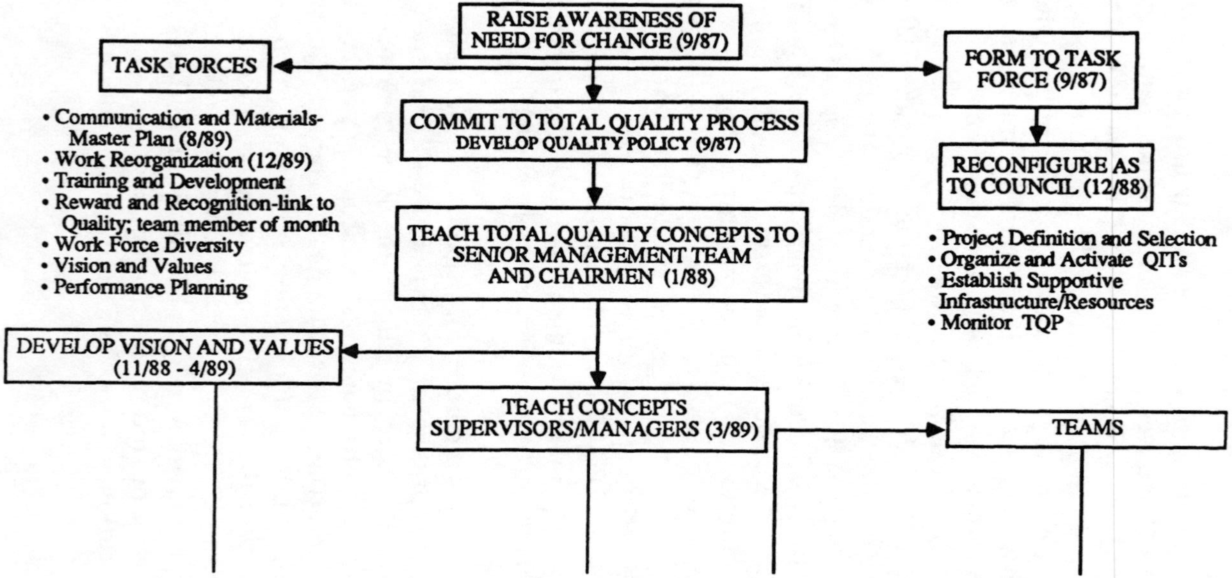

RAISE AWARENESS OF NEED FOR CHANGE (9/87)

FORM TQ TASK FORCE (9/87)

RECONFIGURE AS TQ COUNCIL (12/88)
- Project Definition and Selection
- Organize and Activate QIT's
- Establish Supportive Infrastructure/Resources
- Monitor TQP

COMMIT TO TOTAL QUALITY PROCESS DEVELOP QUALITY POLICY (9/87)

TEACH TOTAL QUALITY CONCEPTS TO SENIOR MANAGEMENT TEAM AND CHAIRMEN (1/88)

TEACH CONCEPTS SUPERVISORS/MANAGERS (3/89)

TEAMS

DEVELOP VISION AND VALUES (11/88 - 4/89)

TASK FORCES
- Communication and Materials-Master Plan (8/89)
- Work Reorganization (12/89)
- Training and Development
- Reward and Recognition-link to Quality; team member of month
- Work Force Diversity
- Vision and Values
- Performance Planning

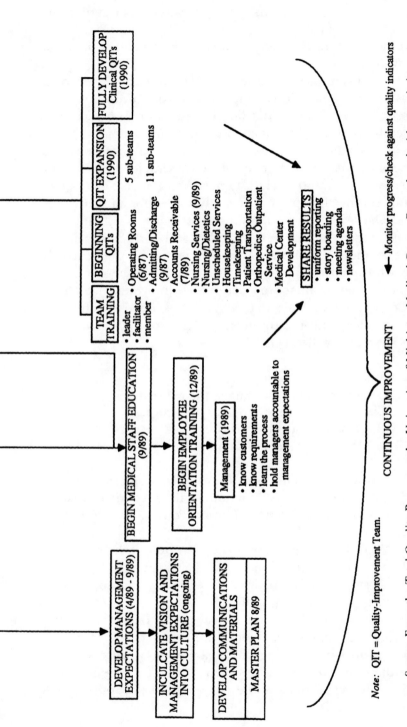

DEVELOP MANAGEMENT EXPECTATIONS (4/89 - 9/89)

INCULCATE VISION AND MANAGEMENT EXPECTATIONS INTO CULTURE (ongoing)

DEVELOP COMMUNICATIONS AND MATERIALS

MASTER PLAN 8/89

BEGIN MEDICAL STAFF EDUCATION (9/89)

BEGIN EMPLOYEE ORIENTATION TRAINING (12/89)

Management (1989)
- know customers
- know requirements
- learn the process
- hold managers accountable to management expectations

TEAM TRAINING
- leader
- facilitator
- member

BEGINNING QITs
- Operating Rooms (6/87)
- Admitting/Discharge (9/87)
- Accounts Receivable (7/89)
- Nursing Services (9/89)
- Nursing/Dietetics
- Unscheduled Services
- Housekeeping
- Timekeeping
- Patient Transportation
- Orthopedics Outpatient Service
- Medical Center Development

QIT EXPANSION (1990)
5 sub-teams

11 sub-teams

FULLY DEVELOP Clinical QITs (1990)

SHARE RESULTS
- uniform reporting
- story boarding
- meeting agenda
- newsletters

CONTINUOUS IMPROVEMENT

→ Monitor progress/check against quality indicators

Note: QIT = Quality-Improvement Team.

Source: From the Total Quality Process at the University of Michigan Medical Center. Reproduced with permission.

materials, training and education, diversity, and other organizationwide issues.

Quality-improvement teams (QITs) are appointed to address specific operational improvement opportunities. QITs
investigate and make specific process improvements. Task
forces, by contrast, investigate organizationwide issues. A QIT
investigating a major process will use such tools as flow charts,
cause-effect diagrams, and Pareto charts to set priorities for
different opportunities. The QIT may then generate other QITs,
to address specific opportunities within the overall process.

The leader of a quality-improvement team should be a
line manager with the responsibility and authority to implement solutions. Quality-improvement teams are the heart and
soul of the quality-improvement process. This is where front-line
employees have a chance to make process improvements. Hospital Corporation of America (1989) has developed a useful strategy to guide quality-improvement teams through their analyses.
This strategy is called FOCUS-PDCA:

> **F**ind a process to improve.
> **O**rganize a team that knows the process.
> **C**larify current knowledge of the process.
> **U**nderstand causes of process variation.
> **S**elect the process improvement.

Florida Power and Light uses similar steps: team, reason
for improvement, current situation, analysis, countermeasures,
results, and standardization (Florida Power and Light, 1990,
p. 22).

After these steps comes the Plan-Do-Check-Act (PDCA)
cycle. Continual improvement can be illustrated as a PDCA
cycle, as shown in Figure 18. This cycle is also known as the
Shewhart cycle (Deming, 1986).

The approach is to go repeatedly through this cycle of
learning and making incremental improvements. The first step,
Plan, includes questioning the capability of a process, posing
hypotheses or theories of how the process could be improved,
and predicting the measurable outcomes if the hypotheses hold

Figure 18. Plan-Do-Check-Act Cycle.

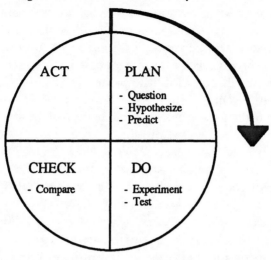

true. The next step, *Do*, includes making changes on an experimental, test, or pilot basis. If possible, changes are made on a small scale first, to avoid major problems if hypotheses are incorrect. In the next step, *Check*, the outcomes of the experiment are verified with comparisons between the measured outcomes and the predictions. Finally, if the hypotheses have proved useful, you *Act* by implementing the changes on a broader scale. If the hypotheses are not useful, you return the experimental unit to the former methods. The same process is repeated for continual improvements.

Establishing and Demonstrating Corporate Leadership for Quality

It may seem obvious to emphasize the importance of leadership's commitment during implementation, but leaders' commitment cannot be emphasized enough. Corporate leaders can demonstrate their commitment to quality in the following ways:

1. *Expressing total quality goals loudly and often.* This is especially important for people in top leadership positions.

2. *Developing and demonstrating personal commitment to quality improvement.* Demonstration of commitment through actions is critically important; otherwise, the total quality process will be viewed as lip service, and not a real corporate change. For example, people in the purchasing department will not adopt the principle of minimizing total cost (rather than minimizing the purchase price) if administrators of the purchasing department continue to demand evidence of lowest purchase price.

3. *Establishing a corporate quality council,* including all corporate officers, physician leaders, nursing leaders, and others, to steer the process. Leadership of the quality-improvement process cannot be delegated effectively.

4. *Appointing a coordinator or facilitator,* who will take corporate responsibility for coordinating training and quality-improvement efforts and monitor progress toward goals.

5. *Committing personal time and effort to attaining quality improvement.* Individual leaders should conduct one or more quality-improvement teams themselves. Managers and staff people watch leaders for cues to what is important. Personal involvement sends a strong message.

6. *Promoting quality actively* in all verbal and written forums. Employees should have no questions about leaders' stated support of quality. Leaders should discuss quality objectives and progress at meetings.

7. *Recognizing, rewarding, and promoting employees* who epitomize quality of services and management.

8. *Publicizing and communicating goals and progress broadly.* This step could include distributing wallet-size cards with values statements for all employees, posting values and goals in prominent locations, and placing articles in the organization's publications.

9. *Integrating quality* into the business planning process.

> *Action Step*: **Personally promote and act in support of quality improvement, every day in every setting. In every meeting, discuss quality and process improvement.**

The most vivid demonstration of quality to an organization occurs when management takes visible actions to identify and meet customers' requirements, especially when there are obvious short-term costs of time, effort, or money. Without action, there will be no meaningful change. Managers' expectations of their subordinates are also a good place to focus quality-improvement behaviors.

Identifying Customers

Quality leaders throughout the world emphasize identifying customers and meeting their requirements as the key step in quality improvement. In healthcare organizations, as we have been saying, the following groups are customers for various services:

Patients. These are the primary consumers of our services and products. One constraint to a broader view of quality in healthcare is the commonly held view that patients cannot evaluate the true quality of the services they receive. That may be true, but they do make judgments about quality, on which they act. Patients can judge their requirements and priorities from their own perspectives. Hospices, for example, developed because patients and their families placed a higher priority on patients' being able to die in a comfortable setting than on heroic surgical and intensive-care efforts.

Physicians. The majority of decisions related to the requirement for healthcare services, as well as the prescription of the types, methods, frequency, and duration of services, are made by physicians. Hence, they are customers for information from many sources and can describe their own requirements.

Nurses. Nurses are major providers of patient care, but they are also the customers of physicians, laboratory and other departments, clerks, and others. Nurses, too, can describe their own requirements and priorities.

Other Healthcare Professionals. Social workers, technicians, and many other professionals deliver care to patients and receive services and information from one another and from suppliers. Each group also has professional standards similar to those established by physicians. Each professional group has requirements for information, equipment, support, and so on, to provide quality patient care and information to physicians and others.

Patients' Families and Friends. These people also must be considered in the equation. Many times, a patient is too ill to judge quality effectively, and these peripheral customers make judgments about quality and whether to use your services in the future. Families and friends can provide valuable insights into the needs of their loved ones, as well as into their own requirements as visitors.

Co-workers. For the majority of activities in a healthcare organization, co-workers are internal customers. Virtually every person in a healthcare organization is a customer of someone else at some time. Moreover, the people performing jobs are the best people to describe the requirements of those jobs. For example, the mailroom clerk can best describe what changes would allow him or her to deliver the mail sooner.

Leaders and Managers. Managers are customers themselves. They receive information as input to their decisions and actions to plan, control, and improve processes. Managers can describe what information they need for planning and coordinating activities throughout the organization.

Professional Associations. Organizations like the JCAHO, professional review organizations, and each association of healthcare professionals have some role in evaluating quality. These organizations develop requirements for accreditation, certification, and approval. To plan changes to meet the requirements, your organization must know what those requirements are.

Payers. For our purposes here, third-party payers are defined to include any individual or organization that pays, directly or indirectly, for healthcare services and products. Examples include employees, employers, unions, insurance companies, and government agencies. Payers evaluate quality, to determine whether they, their members, or their customers are receiving service of acceptable quality and value. It is important to know what information and care payers need, so that accurate and complete bills can be provided the first time.

Determining and Agreeing on Customers' Requirements

Once your external and internal customers have been identified, it is very important to define the valid requirements of each customer. Defining customers' valid requirements is commonly a three-step process. First, determine what the customer perceives as his or her requirements. This can be accomplished only by directly communicating with each customer. Once the requirements are listed, they are assessed. If the customer's initial requirements are perceived by the supplier as inappropriate, there may be a second step — negotiation. The supplier may be able to recommend a better alternative. The third step is agreeing on the requirements and on how they will be met.

The nursing department's supplemental staffing office at the University of Michigan Hospitals (UMH) provides a good example of this process. Historically, head nurses of the inpatient care units could request supplemental staff from either external nursing agencies or from the UMH supplemental staffing office. Most head nurses contracted with external agencies because the internal staffing office did not meet their requirements. When a new manager was appointed for the supplemental staffing office, she adopted a total quality approach. She met individually with her customers, the head nurses, to determine their requirements and priorities. On the basis of their requirements and priorities, new policies and procedures were developed for staff assignment and categories of nurses. The manager continues to meet regularly with the head nurses about their requirements and to provide monthly reports of performance.

Action Step: Begin the process of identifying customers and their valid requirements throughout your organization.

It is helpful to list all external and internal customers and their valid requirements for each product and service of each department. Communicate directly with customers about their requirements. In some cases, it may be appropriate to negotiate requirements.

Action Step: Educate managers to lead forums where employees can brainstorm about external and internal customers for the products, services, and information they provide.

An extension of this approach is to ask each manager to list each of his or her suppliers and to say whether his or her requirements are being met by each supplier. If not, ask for a specific list of requirements that are not being met. This list then serves as an agenda for quality improvement. In most cases, the supplier can improve to meet the customer's requirements, but new requirements can also be negotiated. It may also happen that current performance meets the new requirements.

Customers' requirements may change. Each customer should be asked to discuss any changes. In addition, each supplier should regularly initiate reviews of requirements.

As we have said, it is important to distinguish evolutionary changes (best driven by customers' requirements) from revolutionary changes (best driven by research and product development based on understanding of customers' situations).

Meeting Customers' Requirements

The goal is to meet every valid customer's requirement, every time. Anything less is poor quality. The customer's requirements, of course, may include acceptable tolerances, but once the requirements are agreed to, they must be met every time. Any failure to meet a customer's requirement is an error.

From an operational standpoint, quality objectives can be approached in two ways. The first approach is improvement of quality, or reduction of errors. This approach sets short-term goals for quality improvement. Once a goal is reached, that accomplishment should be celebrated, and a higher goal is then established. In this approach, you can provide positive feedback for improvement, rather than negative feedback for residual errors. The second approach, since the goal is error-free work, makes errors unacceptable. This approach is most useful if the customer's requirements can be reasonably met with current processes. Otherwise, employees will become frustrated with their own inability to accomplish the goal. A useful technique for setting priorities in issues for quality improvement is to consider customers' perceptions of quality, as well as customers' weighting of the relative importance of various issues.

Recent inpatient surveys at the University of Michigan Medical Center indicate that patients base their judgments more on medical care factors than on noncare factors. This may indicate increasing knowledge on the part of patients about important aspects of their care.

Measuring the Cost of Quality

There is some disagreement among quality experts about the relative importance of measuring the cost of quality. This is a key component of Crosby's approach, while Deming and Juran place less emphasis on it.

The total cost of quality includes the costs of quality planning, quality control, quality improvement, and poor-quality output. We believe that healthcare, like other industries, pays a high price for poor quality, particularly as it relates to inadequate communications. Feigenbaum (1987) has estimated that quality-leveraged companies obtain reductions of one-third to one-half in quality costs as compared to their competitors. Crosby (1979) has set that proportion at 15 to 20 percent. The total cost of quality—or, more appropriately, the cost of poor quality—includes such costs and losses as those that follow:

1. Costs associated with giving medications or treatments to the wrong patient.
2. Rework costs of labor, wasted supplies, shipping, and so on. In the healthcare field, an example of rework would be three tries at starting an intravenous line or retaking X rays because of positioning or developing mistakes.
3. Lost labor, equipment time, and supplies on services and products that have to be replaced (for example, radiology or electrocardiogram films, tracings, and reports).
4. Costs of delays. Miscommunication is a common problem that results in delays. Such delays lead to extra labor costs, extended lengths of inpatient stays, lost revenues, and carrying costs of unpaid charges. For example, if a physician requests consultation from a specialist and the results of that consultation are delayed, the patient may remain in the hospital an extra day or longer. One large teaching hospital conducted a detailed clinical audit of medical records for discharged patients and found that over $1.5 million per year was being lost through extended stays resulting from delayed consultations.
5. Lost sales because of dissatisfied patients, physicians, and other customers. This cost is very hard to measure, but it is most important. Loss of the future use of your institution by a patient or a family because of poor service can be huge. Each dissatisfied customer tells approximately nine others, whereas a satisfied customer tells four others. Dissatisfied customers create a ripple effect that is very damaging.
6. Costs of inspection. The time, staff, equipment, and costs of inspection or double-checking for quality are included in the costs of inspection. An example is the large number of first-line supervisors for staff people.
7. Costs of prevention. These represent the engineering and system changes designed and implemented to prevent errors in meeting customers' requirements. Over time, these are the most effective and least expensive functions.

8. Costs of design. Although these are difficult to separate, the additional costs of designing a process that improves quality is also part of the cost of quality.

The key for healthcare organizations is first to reduce the large total costs of poor quality that result from waste, rework, and lost customers and then to shift some of those funds to prevention and design. We recommend calculating the cost of quality, for three reasons. First, estimating the cost of poor quality is an excellent way to gain the attention and support of top management. Second, it is a good way of setting priorities for different quality-improvement projects. Third, reductions in the costs of poor quality are good measures of the effectiveness of quality-improvement projects.

> *Action Step*: **Establish one or more measurable quality-improvement goals for the most important functions of each department, and monitor progress toward quality improvement.**

Cost-Effectiveness of Different Approaches to Quality

There are three different approaches to achieving high-quality output from a system. Good quality-improvement and quality-control processes include a blend of inspection, prevention, and design. Design and prevention should be emphasized as the best approaches to achieving both quality and cost-effectiveness. In some organizations, the attitudes and budgeting related to staff and support costs for prevention and design will have to change. The common attitude minimizes the time and cost for getting a process implemented and gives little consideration to the later costs of an ineffective process.

Inspection. The process of inspection can raise the quality of products or services, but it is costly because it simply removes defective outputs before they reach customers. Costs of inspection, rework, waste, and customer dissatisfaction (if an error is not detected by inspection) are added to the initial cost to produce the service or product. Some amount of inspection will be required, but this is the least desirable approach. The major reason why most healthcare professionals think that increased quality always increases costs is that we have traditionally approached quality improvement through costly inspection.

Prevention. A more effective approach to quality improvement is to prevent errors or problems. This approach requires more initial effort, to identify and eliminate causes of problems, but it is more cost-effective because problems do not recur. For example, when staff are trained to use the same operating definitions and procedures, variations and errors are reduced.

Design. The best approach to producing improved quality is to initially design processes so as to avoid problems. This requires a major initial effort, to anticipate potential uses and problems with a service, product, or process.

Focus on System Improvements

Deming, Juran, Crosby, and other quality experts agree that approximately 85 percent of quality problems and opportunities for improvement relate to changes in systems and processes to produce and deliver services or products. This is the concept of "working smarter." Only 15 percent of improvement potential concerns employees' working harder or more diligently. Therefore, the focus for quality improvement should be systems and processes. Employees' improvement is important in the process because it allows them to work more effectively.

A hypothetical example involving a financial services department will illustrate that system improvements will normally produce greater results than employees' changes alone. The financial services department of a typical large medical center may have several locations, with patient accounts, billing, and collections geographically separated. Problems may include large numbers of records transferred among sections, large duplication costs, delays in obtaining records, delayed mail arrivals, delayed bank deposits, and huge labor costs. To correct these problems, the functions performed, the customers for each function, and the requirements of each customer can be defined to evaluate the current process. Through a change in the physical locations of the functions and filing methods, the requirement for interfunction transportation of records can be virtually eliminated. The result will be substantial and simultaneous improvement in both quality and costs. Without such changes in systems, employees would be very limited in the improvements they could make.

> *Action Step*: **For every identified quality problem, seek improvements in systems and processes first.**

Continual Improvement

Again, all the major quality experts agree that the key to long-term success is the pursuit of continual improvement. This maxim applies to quality, productivity, and any other measure of your organization's performance. Continual improvement is conceptually simple enough, but few organizations effectively use it. To test your organization's status with regard to continual improvement, answer these questions:

1. Are quality and continual improvement on your regular agenda for meetings?
2. Do managers and employees regularly raise ideas to improve quality or productivity?
3. Do managers openly pursue methods of improving quality with their employees?
4. Are employees and managers who propose changes valued and celebrated?
5. If a manager identified a method of improving quality or productivity, would the benefits be made available to the corporation? (Managers commonly try to reallocate benefits within their own areas, and the overall organization may not benefit.)
6. Would a manager who identified a quality improvement

that eliminated staff (or, for that matter, his or her own position) be retained and recognized? (In many institutions, reducing the number of one's staff effectively limits or even reduces one's salary.)

7. After a substantial project has been implemented, do managers continue to seek further improvements? (It is common for managers and staff, after they complete a large project, to relax for a year or so.)

If you answered no to any of these questions, then your current managers are not continually improving to benefit the organization. The Japanese have a term for continual improvement— *kaizen*. According to Imai (1986), the word means not only improvement at work but also "continuing improvement in personal life [and] social life." In the workplace, *kaizen* means "continuing improvement involving everyone—managers and workers alike" (Imai, 1986, p. xx).

Employee Involvement and Training

The single most important approach to improving quality and cost-effectiveness is to involve all employees, physicians, and managers. The people closest to the actual work are the key to both the methods of improving processes and the motivation to improve. Also, circumstances that create adversarial environments must be eliminated.

For widespread quality improvement, managers and employees at all levels must get involved in quality improvement. Nevertheless, it is unreasonable to think that people will automatically understand the principles and practices of total quality. Every employee should receive some level of training related to quality concepts and techniques. More specifically, training targeted to statistical tools and techniques should be provided for quality-improvement teams and other employees. The goal is to get all employees using scientifically oriented problem solving to improve work processes.

Initial Actions for Leaders

This section lists eleven actions that any manager in your organization can take to begin a total quality process in his or her area. This statement assumes that your corporate mission and values statements are already developed, and that managers have been through initial training.

This is an iterative process of investigation, prioritization, action, and improvement. After identifying processes (step 4), you may focus your efforts on one or more processes where there are known major opportunities for improvement. Your initial efforts could be to identify customers, customers' requirements, process capabilities, theories, and actions to realize opportunities. (Chapter Ten explains the following actions in more detail.)

1. Understand and live by the organization's values and management expectations.
2. Develop missions and goals for your department(s). These should be based on the organization's mission and goals, so that departmental and personal goals are aligned with the organization's goals. First list the goals, and then set priorities for them.
3. Demonstrate commitment, sponsorship, and participation for quality improvement. You should visibly live by what you preach.
4. Identify and understand processes within your department(s) and those processes involving other departments. Focus on processes, rather than on departments, to avoid interdepartmental barriers. Look at each process. Can it be simplified or streamlined? Can you reduce the number of steps or people involved?
5. Identify internal and external customers and suppliers for processes.
6. Determine customers' requirements. Measures of performance should be based on those requirements.
7. Understand process capabilities. No matter what you

would like to see happen, the first step is to graph the current capabilities of the processes involved.

8. Encourage ideas and theories of how to improve quality. Normally, the same ideas that improve quality also improve cost-effectiveness.
9. Evaluate and set priorities for opportunities. It is best to use quantitative measures.
10. Take action, if that is in your control. Use the PDCA cycle.
11. Ask for help to start an interdepartmental quality-improvement team. Until managers and staff gain experience with a quality-improvement team, it is a good idea to have a trained facilitator help.

Establishing a total quality process is central to continual improvement of your services, products, and information. The rewards gained from a total quality process are impressive: satisfied and loyal customers, effective systems that make provision of clinical care easier, higher revenues and returns on investments, higher productivity, higher morale, and lower costs.

Chapter Six

Building a Culture
of Continual Improvement

The environment facing healthcare organizations is changing dramatically. Experts have defined this change as a major paradigm shift, encompassing changes in social expectations, as well as in the services and behaviors required of providers. Organizations that are not committed to continual improvement will face major difficulty; the only questions are how soon they will feel the pain, and how they will manage it.

Continual improvement is the objective, not change for change's sake. The most basic question, of course, concerns who defines *improvement*. According to the philosophy of total quality (see Chapter Five), improvement must ultimately be defined by the customers. Even research and education are directed toward improved patient care, although changes in practice may still lie several years ahead.

Continual improvement should apply to all aspects of your organization, including clinical care (surgical practice, medical practice, nursing practice, imaging), operational systems (communication, transportation, financial services), information management and use, and management (including organization to provide services and products, delegation of decision making, employee involvement, and so on).

The concept of continual improvement is one that can be easily supported. Who could possibly be opposed to continual improvement? Yet few organizations have accomplished continual improvement in more than a few areas, and still fewer have created a culture that nurtures continual improvement.

Continual improvement is driven from two perspectives. First, and most important, the external customers of healthcare providers are demanding improved quality and cost control. These external customers include patients, third-party payers, and the businesses and industries that pay directly or indirectly for healthcare services. Second, there is competition among healthcare providers. If one or more organizations become more cost-effective than their competitors, those organizations will gain market share. For example, if patients once go to an outpatient service and are served courteously, with minimal waiting time, they will be unwilling to accept a lower quality of service from similar providers in the future. Customers expect only what you or your competitors lead them to expect, either through service or advertising. If (as has been true for most of the last twenty years) healthcare providers in general offer almost no improvements in service, then customers will have little choice; but if one or more competitors begin to offer improved services and reduced costs, customers will shift away from less cost-effective providers because each customer, on the basis of his or her own definitions and priorities, will decide to select services and products with improved quality and decreased costs. Decision priorities can be easily understood when measures of cost and quality are graphed, as in Figure 19.

Continual improvement is critical to a continuing cycle of improved quality, leading to improved productivity, leading to improved market share, as illustrated in Figure 20. It is very important to understand that process improvements that lead to improved quality also lead to improved efficiency and cost-effectiveness. Continual quality improvement occurs through continual application of the Plan-Do-Check-Act (PDCA) cycle, described in Chapter Five.

Why Continual Improvement Has Not Been Established as a Culture

We are unaware of any healthcare organization that has fully demonstrated a cultural change toward continual improvement, but many organizations are beginning the process and making substantial progress. Some common reasons why orga-

Figure 19. Customer's Priority for Purchase of Services and Products.

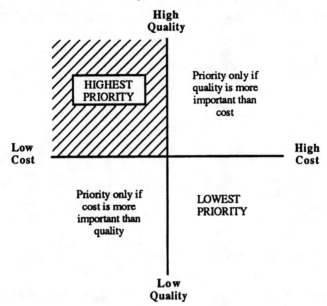

nizations do not undertake continual improvement are discussed in the sections that follow.

No Perceived Need or Urgency for Change. Cost-based reimbursement and slow rates of change among competitors have lulled board members and executives of healthcare organizations into a false sense of security. With little emphasis on customers' expectations, healthcare professionals have determined what they considered appropriate for patient care and service. Clinical care, imaging technologies, and treatment technologies have been changing rapidly, but money has been readily available to buy these technologies. The situation has been easy and comfortable. Why change? There has been little incentive to undertake the risks.

Risk Aversion. Boards, executives, physicians, and others avoid risks whenever possible. They tend to avoid changes unless forced to change. This attitude reflects a crisis orientation and is

Figure 20. Continual Improvement Cycle.

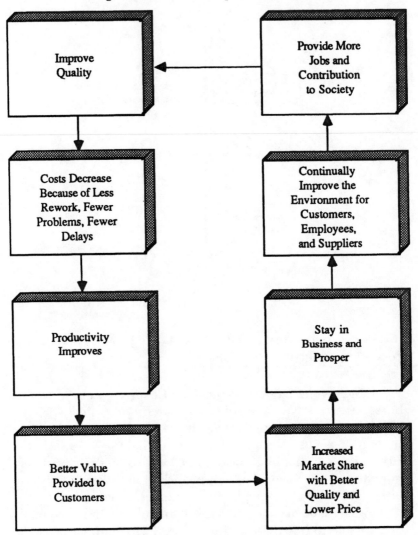

communicated to others through various statements and actions. It is no wonder that physicians and hospitals cling to tradition, continuing, for example, to admit patients the day before minor surgery, rather than performing such procedures on an outpatient basis. Why risk problems, patients' dissatisfaction, and malpractice claims?

The "Standards" Mentality. Boards, executives, and staffs of healthcare organizations have generally subscribed to the notion that there is a single standard of time or resources required for a particular service. This attitude was adopted from U.S. industrial corporations, which themselves have run into trouble from foreign competition. There has been much debate about appropriate standards, and most organizations have not formally implemented any, but the mentality has been that a standard is appropriate and, once reached, needs no improvement. It is common, for example, to find standards or guidelines stating that an error rate (in forms, and so on) of 2 to 5 percent is acceptable. As long as it is acceptable to have an error rate of 5 percent, there is little motivation to improve.

Lack of Understanding of Statistical Variation. The output of any human or machine process will not be constant; it will vary from service to service and product to product. For example, the time to perform a procedure will vary from case to case, even if the same person does exactly the same procedure. Yet managers, staff people, and physicians tend to view outcomes as deterministic (nonvariable) and to make decisions based on single measurements, without considering the sequence of measurements over time. Action is taken when performance deviates from an expected level, even if an employee has done nothing differently, if the deviation is within normal variation, and if the process is stable. Such action is known as tampering and leads to poorer, not better, performance. Lack of statistical understanding causes managers to focus on the wrong topics and questions.

Misconceptions About Problems. As an extension of lack of understanding of statistical variation, workers are often viewed as the source of problems. Nevertheless, approximately 85 percent of all problems result from system or process problems, rather than being caused by incapable or unmotivated employees. Surely, few employees intend to perform poorly; far more improvement can be gained through improvement of the processes used by all employees.

Problems of Focus. Most performance measurements and rewards are based on individual performance. Each person is trying to maximize his or her own achievement and is often unwilling to cooperate or share with fellow workers, especially outside the department. This attitude is counterproductive to group, departmental, and organizational improvement. For example, if two employees are being evaluated on billing goals, both employees will try to maximize their own performance and will focus on procedures that produce the most revenue per hour. Both will avoid difficult or nonbillable activities, even if they are important to the department overall. The same is true among departments. Nursing services may want rooms cleaned more promptly for newly admitted patients, but housekeeping resists because this practice may increase the department's costs, since departments are strictly evaluated on their adherence to budgetary guidelines.

Actions Necessary for Continual Improvement

Management is responsible for achieving continual improvement and must change the organizational culture, develop systems, and create a hospitable environment. Executives of healthcare organizations are responsible for making the changes that will result in continual improvement. This is probably the most important undertaking of the board and corporate officers.

Changes in a corporate culture occur slowly. To change the beliefs, behavior, and assumptions of a group takes time. Managers have conditioned their employees to act in certain ways. Employees must hear about the proposed changes regularly but, more important, they must see managers act in support of those changes. You must begin immediately, but be patient; such behavioral changes take time.

Action Step: **Understand and communicate the need and urgency for change.**

You must first internalize the need to change and develop a vision for the future, as described in Chapter Four. Then you must regularly communicate this need to everyone in your organization through publications, speeches, and, most important, actions.

Action Step: **Focus attention on customers, customers' requirements, and quality.**

If everyone in your organization identifies with external and internal customers and their requirements, there will be much less attention paid to personal and internal topics.

Action Step: **Develop and communicate an understanding of statistical variation.**

If they understand normal statistical variation, managers will ask more appropriate questions, make better decisions, reduce variation, and improve services and products. The easiest way to approach this state of affairs is to change the data on which you and other managers make decisions. For example, before you make a decision, require managers, physicians, and staff people to present a graph of the relevant data, rather than data from a single day, week, or month. Simply by requiring everyone to look at graphs of data, you will help improve decisions. It is much easier to understand variations and trends from graphs than from tables of data.

Action Step: **Provide feedback.**

Provide information to managers and staff members. They want to know how well they are doing. Posting graphs of performance measurements will provide both better under-standing and incentives to improve. One technique is to provide employees with information about your organization, as though they were owners. If you expect employees to act with the incen-tives and pride of owners, treat them as owners.

Action Step: Focus on process improvements.

Process and systems improvements will accomplish about 85 percent of the potential improvements in outputs. Re-member, only in unusual circumstances are people the prob-lem. By focusing on processes, you avoid blaming people, which reduces resistance to change. For example, a number of clerks may be employed to work on bills rejected by third-party payers. Rather than focusing on making these clerks work harder, im-prove the processes for information collection and billing be-fore the bill is sent. This may eliminate the need for the rejection clerks entirely.

Action Step: Focus on group or team improvements, rather than on individual accomplishments.

The organization benefits most from improved overall performance, not from the accomplishments of individuals. Clearly, individuals are important, and you want to commend exemplary individual performance, but only if it contributes to the accomplishments of groups, departments, and the organiza-tion. By looking at overall benefits and costs, you avoid recogniz-ing individual and departmental gains at the expense of the organization.

Action Step: Provide resources for improvement.

Most improvements result from the contributions of many people, often from many departments. For example, im-provement of transportation services for patients will require input from transporters, nurses, physical therapists, other inter-nal and external customers, and managers of the respective areas. Overall, quality improvements will lead to improved cost-effectiveness, but managers must provide staff time and other resources to support education, training, and quality-improvement projects.

> *Action Step*: **Provide recognition and incentives for physicians, managers, and employees who recommend and implement changes.**

Money is important, but so is recognition of individuals and departments. People like to feel that they have contributed and that their contributions are recognized. Examples of non-monetary recognition include complimenting teams and individual employees while making rounds, complimenting people during meetings, using labels or tags so that customers can identify the teams or persons who have helped them, and providing distinctive uniforms. The University of Michigan Hospitals use distinctive uniforms for the door attendants who assist patients as they arrive. These people feel pride, and the patients and visitors appreciate the image and the help.

People have been conditioned for years to be risk-averse, and it will take encouragement and support for them to change. People who suggest and then help to implement changes must be protected and honored because they will face resistance from co-workers and other departments. Care must be taken, however, that the new incentives do not create inappropriate individual or departmental competition.

Fourteen Points for Continual Improvement

The following is a condensation of the fourteen points for management prescribed by Deming, with some healthcare examples. These are very important principles for healthcare managers to understand. According to Deming (1986, p. 23), "The fourteen points are the basis for transformation of American industry. It will not suffice merely to solve problems, big or little. Adoption and action on the fourteen points are a signal that the management intend[s] to stay in business and aim[s] to protect investors and jobs. Such a system formed the basis for lessons for top management in Japan in 1950 and in subsequent years.... The ... points apply anywhere, to small organizations as well as to large ones, to the service industry as well as to manufacturing. They apply to a division within a company."

1. *"Create constancy of purpose for improvement of product and service*, with the aim to become competitive and to stay in business, and to provide jobs" (Deming, 1986, p. 23). Throughout this book, we have emphasized the importance of a common understanding of the mission, vision, values, and goals.

2. *"Adopt the new philosophy.* We are in a new economic age. Western management must awaken to the challenge, must learn their responsibilities, and take on leadership for change" (Deming, 1986, p. 23). The healthcare industry is in a new economic age, with cost and quality controls imposed by third-party payers and external organizations, increased competition among providers, increased customer expectations, and restrictions in education and research funding. Healthcare leaders must recognize the changing environment and its impact on their organizations. For example, let us consider a likely scenario for healthcare providers over the next five to ten years. The first step will be reimbursement of physicians on the basis of a prospective payment system, such as one that uses diagnosis-related groups (DRGs). The second step will be a combined payment for all providers, based on something similar to DRGs. Your philosophy will have to change. How would the relationships of physicians, hospitals, long-term-care institutions, and other providers change? Who would receive the lump-sum payment, and how would it be disbursed?

3. *"Cease dependence on inspection to achieve quality.* Eliminate the need for inspection on a mass basis by building quality into the product in the first place" (Deming, 1986, p. 23). In large part, traditional quality-assurance systems and accreditation reviews have focused on inspection. Other examples of typical mass inspection are double and triple verification of prescriptions in pharmacies to detect errors and comparison of charge slips with medical records to confirm revenues. Inspection may appear to yield higher quality and increase revenues, but the

cost is high in terms of rework and waste. A better approach is to make improvements of process to reduce errors initially.

4. *"End the practice of awarding business on the basis of price tag alone.* Instead, minimize total cost. Move toward a long-term relationship of loyalty and trust" (Deming, 1986, p. 23). It is easy to show that every additional supplier adds variation to services or products. Even if two suppliers are excellent, the differences in their products can lead to additional training, errors, and transactions. Lower purchase prices do not mean that total costs to your organization will be lower. We are all familiar with problems of lowest bidder. The total cost to the institution should be estimated. For example, the University of Michigan Hospitals, Ann Arbor, established a single contract for the large majority of forms used by the hospitals. The quality and standardization of forms was improved, off-site warehouse space was eliminated, time of distribution was reduced, and an on-site print shop was closed. Given the large volume of purchases, the vendor provides on-site representatives to work with managers and staff to meet their requirements. Other vendors' prices for individual forms may be lower, but total costs to the organization have been reduced approximately $280,000 per year.

5. *"Improve constantly and forever the system of production and service* to improve quality and productivity, and thus constantly decrease costs" (Deming, 1986, p. 23). Healthcare organizations cannot afford the status quo; we must continually improve to remain viable. The concept of continual improvement is contrary to traditional concepts of acceptable, constant standards or defect rates.

6. *"Institute training on the job"* (Deming, 1986, p. 23). Training is key to reducing levels of management and to producing more effective employee involvement and self-directed work teams. We must seek out people from our increasingly diverse work force and provide on-the-job training to supplement skills. This is particularly important for the skills of professionals in short supply, such as nurses and allied health professionals.

7. *"Institute leadership.* The aim of supervision should be to help people and machines to do a better job. Supervision

of management is in need of overhaul, as well as supervision of production workers" (Deming, 1986, p. 23). We will address the need for improved leadership in Chapter Twelve. Although many managers are reluctant to admit it, most of the problems and opportunities for improvement are created by managers. Their leadership is necessary to accomplish continual improvement.

8. *"Drive out fear*, so that everyone may work effectively for the company. . . . No one can put in his best performance unless he feels secure" (Deming, 1986, pp. 23, 59). Fear is created in many ways and has a very negative effect on the productivity, creativity, and innovation of employees. The annual appraisal of people, the ranking of teams and divisions, must cease. Have employees who suggest cost-saving ideas been accosted by managers or told that their ideas are not valuable? If someone tries a new idea and it fails, is he or she criticized? If so, then your organization is creating fear among its employees. A common fear among healthcare employees is job loss. Many hospitals and other healthcare organizations have terminated employees to reduce costs. One large metropolitan hospital, for example, terminated nine hundred employees in one year. Among the remaining employees, there is massive fear and lost productivity, which will take years to overcome. Costs must be reduced, but if fear is to be avoided, every possible effort must be made to use attrition, early retirement, and other voluntary methods to reduce the work force.

9. *"Break down barriers between departments*. . . . People in research, design, sales, and production must work as a team, to foresee problems of production and in use that may be encountered with the product or service" (Deming, 1986, p. 24). In most healthcare organizations, it is common for managers or departments to be rewarded for meeting their individual or departmental goals. This practice encourages them to meet the goals, even if by doing so they cause problems elsewhere. For example, limiting or reducing the number of people who transport patients often leads to delays in radiology, physical therapy, nursing, and other departments. Patient transportation has met its budget goals, but the costs of delay, lost productivity, and rework

in other departments may be far greater than the savings in patient transportation. Furthermore, the organization's goal to meet customers' requirements is not met. We must eliminate such barriers between departments if we are to make meaningful process improvements for the organization as a whole. One approach is to make sure that quality- and process-improvement teams include people from all customer and supplier groups. Another relatively new approach to reducing barriers among staff areas is to use the kind of customer-focused centers of excellence that are being formed in many medical centers. For example, a cancer center focusing on the needs of patients may include several professional and support groups that normally do not work together, such as surgeons, internists, psychologists, social workers, nurses, and clinical staff members.

10. *"Eliminate slogans, exhortations, and targets for the work force* asking for zero defects and new levels of productivity. Such exhortations only create adversarial relationships, as the bulk of the causes of low quality and low productivity belong to the system and thus lie beyond the power of the work force" (Deming, 1986, p. 24). The major harm comes from asking people to do something when they have no method of accomplishing the goal. To establish such goals also assumes that employees do not want to do their best, and that they already know how to meet the goals. The first step is to graph actual measurements of quality and performance, to determine the capabilities of the current process. Then address how the process can be changed to improve performance, rather than simply setting some arbitrary goal.

11. *"Eliminate work standards (quotas). . . .eliminate management by objective.* Eliminate management by number, numerical goals. Substitute leadership" (Deming, 1986, pp. 70, 75). Again, managing by objectives or establishing numerical goals when there is no method of accomplishing them is the problem. An inappropriate use of a numerical quota would be to demand that a physical therapy department increase from 4.5 to 6.0 billable hours per day per therapist, with no method for accomplishment of this change. The administrator making the de-

mand, the departmental manager, and the therapists would all be dissatisfied.

12. *"Remove barriers that rob the hourly worker of his right to pride of workmanship.* The responsibility of supervisors must be changed from sheer numbers to quality. . . . Remove barriers that rob people in management and in engineering of their right to pride of workmanship. This means, inter alia, abolishment of the annual or merit rating and of management by objective" (Deming, 1986, p. 24). The role of leaders and managers should be to remove barriers and serve as mentors, coaches, and trainers. For example, physically consolidating the preadmission review, admitting, and patient-account functions or departments is an effective method of eliminating barriers to communication. Furthermore, this reduces waiting time and difficulties for patients being admitted to hospitals or nursing homes.

13. *"Institute a vigorous program of education and self-improvement.* . . . Encourage education and self-improvement for everyone" (Deming, 1986, pp. 24, 86). You must begin to recognize people as assets. Education increases human capital but appears as an expense on an income statement. It must be viewed as an investment. The aim of education is to increase knowledge and understanding, whereas the aim of training is to increase skills for a particular job. Like training, education will be a key to developing a diverse work force, to meet the needs of your patients and other customers.

14. *"Put everybody in the company to work to accomplish the transformation.* The transformation is everybody's job. . . . Take action to accomplish the transformation" (Deming, 1986, pp. 24, 86). It is shortsighted to try to improve quality and cost-effectiveness by using only the ideas of management. Organizations that can stimulate the creativity and innovation of all employees will improve at a much faster rate. Establishing a "quality" department conveys the wrong message unless the goal of that department is strictly to help other managers and staff members also improve quality. If the "quality" department is viewed as the only department responsible for improvements,

you have lost the much larger opportunity for everyone to contribute to quality.

Deming's fourteen points are controversial and represent a major cultural paradigm shift for leaders and managers in the healthcare industry, as well as in other industries. Probably the most controversial point is the elimination of numerical goals for managers and other employees, especially as such goals are related to compensation. If specific targets or goals are used, people try to set the goals low enough so that they can be reached. Once the goals are reached, people consciously or unconsciously do not continue to improve. This applies to all goals: quality, productivity, budgets, and so on.

Continual Improvement: The Future

Continual improvement is clearly here to stay. It is the topic of several national efforts. For example, the National Demonstration Project on Quality Improvement in Health Care is a collaborative effort of over twenty hospitals to investigate the usefulness of industrial quality-improvement methods in healthcare organizations. The project is supported by the John A. Hartford Foundation in New York and is being led by the Harvard Community Health Plan in Boston. The Joint Commission on Accreditation of Healthcare Organizations is also researching major changes in accreditation requirements, focusing on continual improvement.

We are unaware of any healthcare organization that has been able to fully implement all fourteen of Deming's points or to completely change its culture to incorporate continual improvement throughout. Nevertheless, a number of healthcare organizations are making substantial progress. Probably the largest of these is Hospital Corporation of America (Nashville, Tennessee), which has over one hundred hospitals in various stages of training and implementation. Brigham and Women's Hospital (Boston), Harvard Community Health Plan (Boston), NKC Hospitals, Inc. (Louisville, Kentucky), Rush-Presbyterian–St. Luke's Medical Center (Chicago), and University of Michigan Hospitals (Ann Arbor) have also made major progress.

Chapter Seven

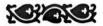

Promoting
Innovation and Creativity

Transformation of your healthcare organization will depend on
greater innovation and creativity. You must unleash the creative interests, knowledge, and skills of the people in your
organization.

If we accept the premise that healthcare will continue to
change at an even faster pace in the 1990s than in the 1980s,
then the issue becomes how we capitalize on, rather than resist,
change. We have noted that the successful healthcare organization will be highly adaptive, creative, and innovative, yet most
large organizations are the antithesis of adaptive organizations.
They tend to be very hierarchical and bureaucratic, and decisions are made in a very traditional manner, far away from the
people providing the services and products. Further, while
adaptability and innovation require risk taking, most managers
in healthcare organizations are risk-averse. By virtue of their
professional training and desire to "cause no harm," they tend to
find it difficult to search for unusual solutions to problems.
Many managers delay making a decision, hoping the problem
will go away. We believe that innovative problem solving is
essential for survival in this time of rapid change. It seems clear
that the culture of risk-averse organizations must be changed to
facilitate risk taking and innovation.

If adaptability and innovation are to be the cornerstones
of success in the future, definitions of these concepts should be
clearly understood by all managers. *Adaptability* is the ability to
adjust to changing circumstances, to be flexible, and to see
change as opportunity. *Creativity* entails developing new ideas or
bringing together existing ideas in original and creative ways.

132

Creativity means finding better ways to do things. An *innovation* is something newly introduced or created. It may be a new method, device, or process of transforming creativity into profit. Systematic innovation is a purposeful and organized search for changes, along with a systematic analysis of the opportunities that such changes may offer for further economic or social innovation. Innovation is the specific tool of entrepreneurs; it is the means by which they exploit change. Entrepreneurs see change as normal and healthy. They search for change, respond to it, and exploit it as an opportunity (Drucker, 1985). The innovator is willing to use personal time and energy to develop ideas beyond expectations.

The term *intrapreneur* was coined by Pinchot (1985) to describe innovators who stay within an organization to introduce new products, processes, or services that enable an organization to profit. Rather than *react* to change, this type of individual uses the entrepreneurial spirit to *shape* change and bring ideas and creations forward. Innovators combine ideas from a variety of sources, embrace change as opportunity, and see problems relative to the whole situation. They refuse to see the past as constraining the future (Kanter, 1983). These ideas benefit the entire organization.

Innovation applies to both evolutionary changes and revolutionary changes. These terms were introduced earlier and will be expanded somewhat here. *Evolutionary changes* occur gradually, with a steady improvement of the service or product over time. These changes are not dramatic at any given time, but over time their total impact can be major. Examples of evolutionary change include improvements and added features of inpatient beds, improved service levels in outpatient clinics, testing with less invasive methods, and improved design of prosthetic devices. If processes are not monitored, however, gradual decreases in service can also occur. Diligence and monitoring are required. Customers and service providers are excellent sources of innovation for evolutionary types of improvements.

Revolutionary changes occur very quickly, with a major and sometimes unpredicted change of the service or product. Exam-

ples of revolutionary change include refrigeration, automobiles, and airplanes. In healthcare institutions, recent examples include the use of microcomputers, coronary bypass surgery, and laser surgery. Innovations leading to revolutionary
change normally occur through research, not through customers' expression of a need for a new service or product. For example, people had been completely unaware that refrigeration,
airplanes, and microcomputers were possible; only after seeing
these products in use did people understand their potential.

To encourage innovation in your organization, you must
be flexible. While you cannot plan for specific innovations, you
can encourage innovation by creating a positive environment
for innovation and supporting research in selected areas. You
must plant the seeds and facilitate employees' innovations. Companies that successfully innovate empower employees to use
corporate resources in ways that cannot always be protected or
justified (Pinchot, 1985).

Achieving Broad Employee Participation

In creative organizations, most of the work force is behav-
ing creatively most of the time. This means that all people on all
fronts, from the finance division to housekeeping to the care
providers, must pursue innovation, look for new products and
services, develop new ways of providing old services, find innovative ways to create and satisfy new markets, and improve
quality and cost-effectiveness. The creative organization is dominated by new ideas that are quickly implemented. This transformed type of organization does not just happen. There must
be a very deliberate effort to facilitate creativity and innovation
at all levels of the organization.

A major problem is that, until recently, many organizations have not considered their employees as having valuable
ideas. These organizations treated most employees as if they had
checked their brains at the employee entrance. They ignored the
creative ideas of the large majority of their employees and
thereby wasted tremendous innovative potential. What are your

personal expectations of employees? Are you creating a successful environment in your organization?

How do you generate creativity? The first step is to review whether ideas are solicited from employees and acted on. In the past, we have overlooked employees as a valuable source of innovative cost-saving ideas. We have looked to managers for cost savings and innovations, instead of to the folks on the front lines. As Kanter (1983, p. 18) points out, "Individuals actually need to count for more, because it is people within the organization who come up with new ideas, develop creative responses and push for change before opportunities disappear or minor irritants turn into catastrophes." Innovations, whether in products, market strategies, technological processes, or work practices, are designed not by machines but by people. After years of telling corporate citizens to trust the system, many companies today must relearn instead to "trust their people and encourage them to use neglected creative capacities in order to tap the most potent economic stimulus of all—idea power" (Kanter, 1983, p. 51).

This "idea power" is an essential concept in healthcare and in all other industries as well. Involving the employees in developing creative approaches to the changing environment may mean the difference between success and failure for an organization. We must tip the hierarchical system upside down, give decision-making power for improvement to employees, and find new ways to stimulate everyone to participate in idea generation. Remember, you must personally support and encourage innovation. Innovation will not be sustained unless leaders support and model creative behaviors.

Action Step: Teach people visualization skills.

Try leading a visualization session with your staff. First, do deep-breathing exercises to achieve a relaxed state, and then use visualization to set a goal, the way athletes use visualization by imagining themselves crossing the finish line and winning the race. Create a clear picture of your problem, imagine the variety of barriers, and think about how to overcome each of them.

Focus mentally on your idea often, and continue to explore and shape it. Finally, give positive energy to your idea.

When you reach a mental impasse, follow deBono's (1970) idea of switching from vertical thinking to lateral thinking: swing your thinking around, and see the problem from a new angle. Instead of focusing on the department or other organizational unit, focus on the process, which crosses multiple organizational borders. (This was discussed in relation to quality. improvement in Chapter Five.)

Another suggestion is to teach your people to write down a problem they are struggling with and post it in places where they can see it when their minds are refreshed: on the bathroom mirror, the refrigerator door, or the office telephone. Sooner or later, ideas will flow that will facilitate problem resolution. There is no one best way to do things. In large organizations, multiple approaches to innovation should be pursued.

Setting Expectations

Enhancing creativity in a traditionally oriented organization is not easy. It requires a change in organizational priorities, so that each person, from the front lines to the boardroom, knows that creativity and innovation are basic expectations. If you want ideas, you must solicit and act on them quickly. Many companies that have been successful in enhancing innovation have changed performance criteria for managers to include recording the number of things they have changed in a year; the number of new programs, processes, or services that have been initiated in their divisions; or the number of outdated services that have been deleted.

To enhance creativity in an organization, encourage key managers to develop the essential skills — a composite of style, intuition, and experience — that lead to a creative new method of problem solving. When managers lead the effort, employees know that their ideas are welcome and important and will be acted on. Townsend (1984) suggests training foremen to meet with workers in idea sessions and giving them the authority, without further approval, to try ideas costing up to $150.00. This shows your level of commitment to making things happen.

Drucker (1985) feels that there is only one way to make innovation attractive to managers: a systematic policy of abandoning not only whatever is outworn, obsolete, and no longer productive but also the mistakes, failures, and misdirections of effort. He further suggests that every product, process, and service be put on trial for its life every three years. One could ask such serious questions as "Would we go into this product, this market, this distribution channel, this technology, now?" If the answer is no, then the question becomes "What do we have to do to stop wasting resources on these efforts?" The training and orientation of managers must be based on the concept of teaching them to continually ask questions. The distinctive role of leadership (in a volatile environment, especially) is the quest for "know why" ahead of "know how" (Bennis and Nanus, 1985).

Recruit managers with creative abilities, and nurture them. Protect them, so that they will take analyzed risks and avoid the "Ready, aim, aim, aim" philosophy so prevalent in healthcare. Another key is to give freedom to your staff. Do not build in too much direction, supervision, or reporting. Visibly reward those who seek to solve problems. For example, an employee suggestion program can provide cash rewards for cost-reducing or revenue-enhancing suggestions.

Creating a Nurturing Environment

In Chapter Five, we discussed the importance of building employees' commitment to your mission and goals. Commitment will also help you build creative energy into the organization that will nurture intrapreneurs. For many years, it was necessary for a person who had entrepreneurial desires to leave the organization and strike out on his or her own to find the freedom to follow up on ideas. Gifford Pinchot III was the first to suggest that creative people can be nurtured and supported and allowed to stay in the organization, so that both parties could profit. Pinchot (1985, p. xiii) suggests five steps for enhancing your organization's chances for successful movement toward innovation:

1. Clearly state your vision of the company's future so that intrapreneurs can work on creating innovation that relates to the strategy for the company.
2. Look at every level for intrapreneurs with ideas — not just for ideas alone; an idea without someone passionate about it is sterile.
3. Replace red tape with responsibility.
4. Reward intrapreneurs with new career paths that fit their needs.
5. Advise managers that in the game of musical chairs caused by the removal of layers of unnecessary management, safety of a sort as well as the greatest opportunity lies in becoming an intrapreneur.

Another approach to encouraging innovation is to transfer employees and managers among different departments and thereby broaden their understanding of the organization and its customers. Employees need to think of success in new ways and to see lateral movement in the organization (as well as upward movement) as progress. Many progressive organizations now pay employees more when they learn new skills, such as budgeting, planning, and staffing and scheduling. These skills then promote creativity on quality-improvement teams.

Promoting the Concept of Changing from Within

It is crucial, when you are moving toward a more creative organization, that you set up a structure that will help rather than hinder change. All barriers that preclude innovation must be removed. As a leader, you can begin the process by modeling supportive behaviors. When you are struggling with a management problem, go out into the organization and ask employees for suggestions and solutions. Then follow up on the suggestions and give credit where credit is due.

One note of caution: before you approach employees, make sure you understand the problem completely. Many problems are difficult to solve because they are ill defined. Keep in mind that there is no one right or wrong way to solve a problem; be open to a variety of solutions. Think about combining old things in new ways as you search for alternatives. One exercise that illustrates this concept is to think of as many uses of something as you can. Take the standard paper clip, and think of all the potential uses for this device. Perhaps you thought of using it to hold clothes on a hanger or fastening loose keys together, or using it as a small screwdriver. How about using it as a book mark, or for tying dried flowers together in an arrangement?

Such thinking in analogies was the same type of technique used by engineers at the National Aeronautics and Space Administration to find substitutes for zippers and buttons. The group was trying to find a way for astronauts to manipulate fastening devices while wearing heavy gloves. The use of solutions that work in other applications reflects one concept related to analogies—finding correspondences between dissimilar things. Teach your staff to use this and other creative problem-solving techniques.

Help employees use alternate thinking because curiosity produces new ideas. Ask people to think of what they know from other fields that could be applied to healthcare. Make creativity and innovation fun. Use separate times and places, away from everyday activities, to stimulate people. Remind them of the golux from James Thurber's (1950) book, *The 13 Clocks*. The golux always turned ideas upside down and backwards to find a solution.

Encourage people to daydream creatively. Many major breakthroughs have occurred when people used daydreaming and fantasy. Peter Ueberroth said that this was the technique he used to make the Los Angeles Olympics of 1984 one of the most profitable ever; he was named *Time* magazine's Man of the Year for his success with the Olympics (Ajemian, 1985).

Getting Started

We know that organizations are designed to seek a steady state and exhibit the characteristics of inertia, resistance to change, and maintaining the status quo. The goal is to achieve a steady state trending upward, not laterally or downward. Therefore, you need to assess your organization and figure out where you are in regard to innovative practices.

> *Action Step*: **Complete an audit of the amount of innovative activity occurring in your organization. Ask three questions: Do your employees have degrees of freedom to do their jobs the way they think they should be done, or do they have to continually seek permission? How long does it take to implement a new idea? What rewards are there for innovators?**

If the results of your audit do not match your expectations, there are several steps you can take. First, there must be a clear message from the top of the organization, supported by all managers, that ideas are wanted and will be acted on. Second, if no reward system exists, one should be created. It also must be communicated broadly that it is okay to fail; not all ideas will have positive payoffs. Third, there must be a climate of encouragement, so that employees will learn to think more creatively. Time for the use of creative daydreaming techniques, to imagine a better way of doing things, must be set aside, as well as time to strategize on how to make the imagined changes. This is a difficult management position in an environment of financial constraints.

Be on the lookout for individuals who seem to see problems as opportunities and are open-minded about change. These are the kinds of individuals who can help your organization become more adaptable. There are several characteristics that innovators seem to share. They see problems as opportunities for innovation and welcome the challenge. They have an intuitive ability to identify pieces of a solution that work in other settings and adapt them to healthcare. They keep an open mind in problem solving and remain flexible enough to modify an approach in the face of changing circumstances. They manage to deflect the predictable discouragement and constant potential for failure cited by peers who simply do not share their wisdom (D'Aquila, 1988). Keep these concepts in mind as you search for those who can help you. Once you have identified a cadre of people, set up a time for them to come together and share their ideas. Review the characteristics list at your first meeting, and ask for comments on how to teach these skills to employees. If the time frame to implement new ideas is too long, use your group of innovators to brainstorm how the process can be shortened to help jump-start innovative concepts.

> *Action Step*: **Send out a call for innovative ideas, and act as a sponsor, working with intrapreneurs until projects are completed, to stimulate intrapreneurship. When success is firmly in hand, showcase results and send out another call for project proposals.**

At the University of Michigan Medical Center, an innovation program was pilot tested in nursing services. A call for ideas, sent to every nurse, resulted in several ideas. Mentors sponsored the most promising ones by coaching the innovators and removing barriers. The successful implementation of numerous ideas then served as a basis for expansion of the innovation program to the whole organization.

As managers gain experience in sponsoring projects, delegate the sponsorship of later projects to an ever increasing number of managers. Former intrapreneurs may also make wonderful sponsors because they know the ropes of business-plan development and implementation; chances are that they have had lots of practice recognizing and dealing with potential barriers.

Another useful way of promoting innovation is to expect every manager to encourage it. If performance plans are used, one approach is to include expectations for innovation in every manager's plan. The expectation is that the manager will actively seek and support innovation projects. 3M has a corporate expectation that substantial percentages of each division's annual income will be from products introduced during the previous three years.

Consider using a series of focused meetings to generate ideas. In phase one, you creatively brainstorm and fully explore problems and opportunities. As in any other brainstorming process, do not judge ideas as correct or incorrect. Every idea is listed and framed for future evaluation, and all judgment is suspended.

Phase two becomes the solution-generating phase. Again, use brainstorming to list as many divergent solutions as possible.

In phase three, convergent thinking occurs. Which of the ideas is most effective? Will it produce the desired results? Is the concept sound? Will it represent an improvement over current practice? Is timing appropriate? Is the idea feasible? Will it work? Is it compatible with your mission and goals? Is this the right time? How much will the innovation cost? Analysis becomes more detailed in this phase. The result is a business plan suitable for management to use for a decision. An sample outline of a business plan is given in Chapter Eleven.

Phase four is for planned implementation. The team now needs to look at barriers and obstacles to implementation and develop an action plan.

Let's take an example: Should your organization develop an ambulatory satellite clinic? In phase one, the problem is explored. What populations should be served? What advantages does building a clinic have? What are the objectives? What (if any) other ventures could better meet the objectives? Are the objectives rational? What types of clinics should be offered, in terms of specialties or primary care? Answer these questions: who, what, when, where, and (most important) why?

In phase two of this example, you use brainstorming to review the project from many viewpoints, generating as many concepts as possible related to establishing a satellite clinic. Expand on who, what, why, when, and where. What different approaches could you use? How will your medical staff view these satellite clinics?

In phase three, you converge on the approach and evaluate alternatives. Does your mission support both primary and specialty clinic development? What are the minimum facilities and equipment required? How many hours per day will the clinic be open? Will reimbursement support the concept? What is the return on investment? The staff should reduce the free-wheeling ideas of phases one and two and evaluate a few alternatives. This phase will result in one or more business plans.

In phase four, you work the implementation through. Use creative brainstorming to elicit ideas, and then develop your final action plan. Be sure to include actions that will communicate and build support for the project in the communities involved and among your medical staff, businesses, and employees.

When you begin to use these techniques, your staff will see them as valid ways to solve problems, and creativity will become a way of life. A major benefit of this approach is that the participation of staff members leads to commitment and buy-in, which will help make the project successful.

Funding Innovation

Innovation is a key to future success; it is an investment in the future. Setting aside dollars to develop and reward ideas shows that you are serious about innovation.

> *Action Step*: **Set up a venture-capital pool that any unit with a good idea for a new program can apply for. Structure the pool so that it becomes replenished as projects pay off. A second way you can invest in ideas is to set time aside for processing ideas and reducing potential barriers. Arrange time for employees to learn about and actually use visioning skills to imagine their innovations and any barriers that may impede prog-**

ress. Lead "what if" scenarios with your staff, to get the creative juices flowing.

At the University of Michigan Hospitals, the chief executive officer established an innovation fund, to provide each of three line executives with $1 million for beginning new programs that offered high potential returns on investment. Returns from programs will replenish the fund and pay for future innovations. John Hopkins University formed Triad Investors Corporation, to facilitate the transfer of technology from the laboratory to the marketplace. About eighty large corporations have been invited to invest, in the hope of raising $10 to $30 million (Dine, 1989).

Eliminating Barriers to Innovation

Unfortunately, there are many barriers to creating an innovative climate. They must be identified and removed. The most common barrier is requiring too many approvals before a project or idea is officially blessed. The farther up the ladder the decision must be made, the less chance there is for the completion of an idea. H. Ross Perot, the successful entrepreneur who founded Electronic Data Systems (EDS) and then sold it to the General Motors (GM) Corporation, said, "The first E.D.S.er to see a snake kills it. At G.M. the first person to see a snake calls a consultant who knows a lot about snakes, then they form a committee on snakes and talk about it for a year [and] then maybe something happens" (Perot, 1988, p. 4A). You must free your managers and supervisors to make decisions on the front lines. Develop the policy that the first person to have an idea will know how to get permission to implement it. Encourage pilot projects for testing concepts; Peters (1987) calls this investing in small starts.

Obviously, the move to establish a creative environment presents a dilemma with respect to time and budget. On the one hand, we would like to give employees time to work on innovative ideas; on the other, with more stringent reimbursement limits, there is not enough money to earmark the resources for innovation. Employees need to learn how to set new priorities for innovation by deleting things from their "to do" lists that do not have potential or are no longer needed.

One serious barrier to innovation is to purposely or inadvertently punish someone who has tried a new idea that did not work. If the person is criticized in any way for failure, that person and others will be hesitant to suggest ideas in the future.

Another serious barrier is that in most organizations there are far more idea stoppers than idea supporters. For some reason, we are much more apt to reject people's ideas than to support them. There is a language that people use, without even thinking of the consequences. This language stops the flow of ideas: "That won't work here." "We tried that a few years ago, and it didn't work." "That's not the way we do things here." "Your approach is too academic." Have you ever heard this language in your organization, or perhaps used it yourself? Think of how many good ideas you may have stifled!

> *Action Step*: **Make sure you do not fall into the trap of suppressing ideas. When people suggest ideas, help them flesh out the details. See what potential a concept has before discarding it. Show supportive behavior when people bring ideas forward. Help them think about implementation strategies.**

Innovative companies provide the freedom to act, which arouses the desire to act (Kanter, 1983).

Another common barrier is studying an idea to death, or "paralysis by analysis." Too much study produces inertia. Innovation is unpredictable and occurs through the pursuit of constant experimentation, which we must encourage. Urge employees to ask "what if" questions related to their work.

If you are truly interested in generating ideas with payoffs, there are some phrases that should become part of the language used in your organization: "Tell me more about how you think that idea can be implemented." "How can this idea be used by our organization?" Teach your staff to ask "how" questions: "How can we increase innovation and creativity? Improve our services? Foster cross-departmental ideas? Develop and reward creative ideas? Communicate or spread thoughts and ideas? Implement creative ideas?" Use creative discussion to answer these questions. Also use "wish list" development to get creative juices flowing: "I wish we were rewarded for good ideas." "I wish money were no object." "I wish I could. . . ." "I wish we could. . . ." Then have the staff explore why things *cannot* be done. Creative approaches, such as lotteries, have been able to raise large sums of money for state governments and churches, so why not for healthcare organizations?

The concept, as we have been saying, is to create a supportive environment, where people feel free to bring their ideas forward. Another way to reduce the time between suggestion and implementation is to create a team in each department whose role is to review ideas and work out how to implement them.

> *Action Step*: **Create time at staff meetings when new ideas can be presented and discussed and plans can be made for implementation.**

Evaluate individuals' work loads, and set new priorities. Stop performing outdated activities.

> *Action Step*: **In your company newsletter, list all new ideas that have been implemented in the organization, along with the originators' names and any rewards.**

> *Action Step*: **Review all relevant literature and information about healthcare innovations, as well as about innovations in other fields, so that new applications can be explored.**

The Health Care Forum sponsors an annual catalogue of innovations. Each year, the forum asks readers to submit innovations from the simple addition of a service to changes made in connection with major restructurings or mergers. In the 1988 edition, for example, 101 innovative ideas are written up (Healthcare Forum, 1988).

> *Action Step*: **Send copies of *The Innovators Catalog* or similar documents to your line managers for discussion at departmental meetings, to stimulate innovative thinking. Hearing about others' ideas may spark creativity. Sponsor brown-bag lunches, where people can come to share.**

> *Action Step*: **Read about innovative companies, such as 3M, Hewlett-Packard, AT&T, and Wal-Mart. Learn the strategies they have used to enhance creativity and innovation.**

> *Action Step*: **Nurture all creative ideas that people bring forward.**

Innovation should become a way of life for all employees in your organization. Break down barriers that have stifled creative ideas and enthusiasm. The energy you may unleash can help you keep moving ahead during the change process. Innovation can involve anything your organization does, including the way you organize and conduct work.

Chapter Eight

Reorganizing the Way
People Work and Interact

While most healthcare organizations in the United States have reorganized to some extent in the past decade, few of those reorganizations, even major ones, have significantly affected the way work is accomplished. In most cases, organizational entities were established, consolidated, or eliminated. While the top layers changed, the authority or responsibility of employees did not, nor, in most cases, did reorganization reduce any cross-departmental barriers that were preventing effective work strategies. Decision making continued to be centralized in management ranks. Managers continued to function as directors, controllers, and evaluators, rather than functioning as planners, coaches, counselors, and mentors.

The goals of work reorganization are to change the structure and the way we work to improve how we meet organizational goals. This includes improving the performance of the organization and improving the environment for customers, employees, and suppliers. We want to meet our customers' requirements in the most timely and cost-effective manner possible. Therefore, we must consider such concepts as reducing layers of hierarchy, reducing requirements for communication, increasing employees' involvement and empowerment, and encouraging contributions from all employees. This transformation is based on changed roles, responsibilities, authority, and behavior of managers and employees and requires new relationships between managers and staff people. Leaders must establish and demonstrate new behaviors and serve as role models and mentors for the change process.

148

Background and Definitions

Traditionally, management's job has been seen primarily as control of such resources as time, money, materials, and people. Leaders, however, know that the more they control others, the less likely it is that people will excel. Leaders do not control; they enable others to act (Kouzes and Posner, 1987). As managers, we become more powerful as we build the power of those below us in the organization.

Transformational leaders have been characterized as charismatic, inspirational, able to stimulate others intellectually, and capable of showing individualized consideration (Bass, 1985). This type of leadership is helpful in trying to reorganize the way work is accomplished and the way people relate in an organization. For Naisbitt and Aburdene (1985), the big challenge in the 1980s was retraining managers to deal with changes in the work force. We seem to have made very little progress in dealing with the challenge of an increasingly diverse work force.

For most of the history of the industrial age in America, we have had more potential workers than jobs, and managers have essentially operated in a buyer's market. Demographics are changing dramatically, however, and we must use a new focus to deal with the massive personnel shortages that will face us in the years ahead (Johnston and Packer, 1987). According to Naisbitt and Aburdene (1985), thirty years ago the average worker was a white male with a wife and children. He worked full time, usually in a factory but sometimes in an office, and belonged to a union or would join one. He was about forty and would retire at sixty-five. He was motivated by job security and steady pay. Today, the average worker is a thirty-four-year-old baby boomer with two children and a working spouse. He or she expects to work past retirement because of inadequacies in the Social Security System. This worker does not belong to a union and would not consider joining one. He or she is willing to accept risk in exchange for the possibility of being rewarded for superior performance and is likely to have some sort of flexible work schedule or would prefer one.

More and more women are working today. White males now make up only 46 percent of the work force, and within a few short years, the U.S. Department of Labor (1988) predicts, 85 percent of the people entering the work force will be minorities and women. Because women will make up a larger proportion of the work force (by the year 2000, women will constitute 47 percent), you may need to make changes in your organization. You must manage diversity if you hope to compete effectively in the future.

The corporate environment must be conducive to everyone's growth. Education and training must allow people to confront and overcome the prejudices and assumptions that set up barriers to effectiveness. Perhaps more important, we must listen to the needs of employees, in order to empower them to help us meet corporate goals and objectives. The days of believing that we know what employees need to be successful are over. As our environments become more diverse, we must enhance our listening skills.

We recommend a process of exploring attitudes and behaviors and mapping where you are. Then, you need to develop a plan, to see where you want to go. You need to strengthen the participation of your employees. Some would say we need to transform the corporation from a top-down bureaucracy to a network where everyone learns from everyone else (Naisbitt and Aburdene, 1985). Many organizations are seeking employees' input because they have recognized that people are their most important asset.

There are many ways to enhance employees' involvement. One way is through the effective use of teams, workers and managers who meet periodically to share information and solve problems. Participants must feel a sense of loyalty and commitment. Team building means taking deliberate action to identify and remove barriers, replacing unsound behavior with the kind that can lead to superior performance. Effective teamwork can enhance productivity, creativity, and satisfaction among employees. It can enhance harmony in the organization and lead to a better understanding between employees and managers. Team building in an organization can also reduce the "we-they" division from which many organizations suffer. Motivated employees undertake even routine jobs creatively and become candidates for greater responsibility and productivity (Bradford and Cohen, 1984). Team-building efforts are not a quick-fix strategy for an organization, however. Implementation requires a major change in the beliefs and norms held by the members of the organization.

Many new programs developed to improve corporations fail, not because the programs are unsound but because of resistance to change. When you are contemplating a major shift, you need to keep in mind that successful organizational improvements have certain characteristics (Tichy and Nisberg, 1976):

1. They are purposeful and goal-directed. There are relatively explicit goals and directions toward which the program is aimed.
2. Form follows function. The program is organized, and resources are allocated, on the basis of tasks to be performed, not according to formal authority or power requirements.
3. Decisions are based on the location of relevant information, not on roles in the hierarchy. Determine where decisions are made. Include expert resources throughout your organization to solve problems.
4. Program designers pay explicit attention to the organizational context.

The successful manager will establish a climate for change, where the purpose is made clear and information about the consequences of change is shared in advance and planned for. For employees' involvement, it is not enough to be a visionary leader and lay out a new plan; you must also have a vision strong enough, and an action plan comprehensive enough, to overcome resistance. You must develop a group of sponsors to assist with the formulation and implementation of the plan. Many efforts at involving employees (such as quality circles and the "quality of work life" programs) have failed or received mixed reviews because they were implemented with a short-term focus. When problems arose, there was no sponsor to put the train back on the track, and doubting Thomases could say, "I told you so." Major changes in employees' involvement cannot occur without managers' commitment and involvement. Many of the failed programs ignored such commitment.

Part of the reason for failure is that the culture of an organization must change to facilitate employees' involvement, and a new organizational culture is difficult to build. It is a time-consuming effort that requires patience and energy. Changing the belief system of key stakeholders is a formidable task. According to Bice (1987, p. 447), "Large-scale cultural change is not for everyone. Without [the CEO's] continual involvement and endorsement and without a clear and substantive understanding of the magnitude of the task, any attempt at transformation is bound to fail." A former boss of ours, and CEO at the University of Nebraska Medical Center, C. Edward Schwartz, used to say that changing a health center was similar to turning a battleship around: the captain charts a new course and steers the wheel, but it takes a long, long time to see results.

The New Paradigm of Work

Building a new culture includes creating a vision that includes a new paradigm of work. This paradigm has been described in the current literature, and many organizational design specialists predict that this new model will replace the old system, which has been characterized by authoritarian management and extreme division of labor (Hoerr, Pollack, and Whiteside, 1986). Historically, corporations have relied on control from the top to achieve results. The new model relies on developing employees' commitment (Walton, 1986). The control-oriented paradigm assumes that organizations can best get people to perform their tasks through close supervision and never-ending lists of rules and regulations. The involvement approach takes a different perspective: that workers can figure out the right thing to do if they are given a macro view, organizational goals and objectives, proper training, liberal information, and a two-way communication flow that keeps them informed about progress and any changes in direction. The contrast of the two paradigms is summarized in the following comparison, where the control-oriented paradigm is characterized on the left and the new paradigm is shown on the right:

Control over employees	Empowered employees
Bureaucratic design	Open systems
Individual focus	Team focus
Adversarial management	Atmosphere of trust
Top-down decisions	Decisions on the front lines
Employees seen as expendable	Employees seen as assets

Gitlow and Gitlow (1987, p. 4) explain why we need a new paradigm:

> American industry, once the most productive in the world, has taken a back seat to Japanese industry and cannot produce quality goods and compete in the marketplace. Why? American management is adrift at sea without a rudder or a sail. It doesn't know how to get back on course. It may not even realize that it is off course. U.S. industry doesn't know how to regain its competitive position. American management must realize that we are all in a new economic age, one dominated by the production of quality goods and services at low price rather than mass production of lower quality products. If American managers are to steer their corporate ships, they need to transform their style of management.

Much of the Japanese miracle is due to enhanced teamwork. We know that employees' performance has a tremendous impact on the success of the organization, and so to make progress, you need to develop a vision of what method will work best in your organization. To create an environment for learning and growth, you will need to be a strong advocate for the vision. Start by forming relationships with people at all levels that encourage openness, responsibility, and commitment (Block, 1987).

The goal is to move toward corporate synergy, a process in which cooperation and collaboration yield a product that is greater than the sum of its parts. Synergistic environments reduce conflict and divisiveness.

To begin the visioning process, you should consider the six prerequisites for a good job, which can be the basis of your plan (Thorsrud, 1972):

1. The need for the content of a job to be reasonably demanding of the worker, in terms other than sheer endurance, and yet to provide some variety but not necessarily novelty
2. The worker's need to be able to learn on the job and continue learning
3. The need for some minimal area of decision making that the individual can call his or her own
4. The need for some minimal degree of social support and recognition in the workplace
5. The need for the individual to be able to relate what he or she does and produces to his or her social life
6. The worker's need to feel that the job leads to some sort of desirable future, not necessarily promotion (when employees realize that their goals and management's goals are similar, it enhances cooperation)

Some minor steps can be taken to begin the process of fostering cooperation. The first step may be to initiate an open forum where the CEO can improve communications across the organization. This should begin as a question-and-answer forum. Not all questions will need to be answered at each session, but there must be a method for getting the questioner's name, to provide a correct answer at some time in the future. If the question is of major importance to the institution, feedback to the whole organization can occur through the organization's newspaper or some other communication device. At these meetings, it is important for the CEO to recognize and encourage ongoing interactions and examples of involvement among employees. The CEO must serve as a role model for the cooperative style you are trying to move toward. Introducing managers at the start and involving them in the meetings says loudly that team-work and a cooperative manner are valued.

> *Action Step*: **Begin open employee forums with the chief executive and chief operating officer, to elicit and answer employees' questions and concerns.**

At the University of Michigan Hospitals, the CEO has been holding open employee meetings every four months for eight years. Meetings are held at different hours of the day, so that employees from all shifts can attend. At these meetings, the CEO briefly describes progress and new organizational plans and then opens the meeting to questions about any subject of interest to employees. These meetings have been effective in communicating with employees and identifying their concerns. If information to answer a question is not immediately available, the CEO asks other managers in the audience for assistance. If no one can answer, after the meeting the CEO follows up with the individual who asked the question. If the question is judged to be of general interest, an answer to the question is published for general distribution. If not, the questioner receives a personal response.

The next step is to spread the concept of openness to other levels of the organization, by encouraging other corporate officers to initiate breakfast or lunch meetings, which begin with questions. As groups mature, they can move on to discussions of institutional problems and, finally, to development of plans for change. The goal is to begin to share the vision of increased involvement and get feedback on concepts. Sponsorship for future changes will be much easier to achieve once goals are clear to all work groups. There will still be resisters, but the support base will be broadened. As groups mature even more, they can be used to develop task lists that will bring about necessary changes.

Another strategy for unfreezing attitudes is to begin discussing the benefits that team methods offer over old methods. Allowing employees to catch the vision, as well as participate in identifying barriers that may prevent implementation, can be an empowering strategy.

Management by Specialist

To understand the evolution of management styles, it is useful to review the history of management. Frederick Taylor is often called the father of scientific management, and his methods are still broadly used today in the United States.

Scientific management is a system of "management by specialist." The manager formulates the rules and standards, and the worker follows them. This was a viable method of management when the average worker had a third- or fourth-grade education, and when thinking and communication were not expected or necessary. A serious shortcoming of the Taylor method, however, is that it fails to recognize the increasing educational level of the average employee, the need for personal satisfaction, and the creative potential that each employee brings to the job. Thinking that changes in work process are best made by the manager, rather than by the person doing the work, is shortsighted. In an era when competition requires innovation and creativity at all levels in the organization, we need a system of organization that will recognize the contribution each worker can make. Many studies show that the people who can make the most significant changes are those who do the work or those who are the customers for whom the product is developed or the service provided.

In today's environment, with global competition and a whole new set of highly educated workers looking for job satisfaction and autonomy, a new method of management is essential. The time has come for our workers to be able to use their brains as well as their hands in carrying out their job responsibilities.

One fairly radical method of work reorganization is the concept of self-directed work teams. In the early 1950s, the concept of self-directed work teams was derived from sociotechnical systems (STS) theory (developed at the Tavistock Institute of Human Relations, London), through a series of group experiments that originated in the British coal-mining industry (Trist and Bamforth, 1951). STS is a high-level management approach to improving any work process in a manufacturing or service organization. Procter & Gamble began using the approach in 1969, and both Volvo and General Motors have used STS to radically change the way cars are manufactured.

STS management gets its name from the way it integrates people's production or technical requirements with their organizational or social requirements. Employee involvement and organizational design are key principles, but each of the two major subsystems is optimized; one does not succeed at the expense of the other (Taylor and Asodorian, 1985).

There have been many examples of success in the thirty years since STS research began. Corporations using these methods have seen employees derive satisfaction from doing their jobs well and from participating in projects or reaching goals. There is also satisfaction in being recognized by one's peers for a job well done. This approach is being proved all across the country. Successful companies that have moved to this form of management include Xerox, Honeywell, Procter & Gamble, Digital Equipment Corporation, General Motors, and Ford. They have all realized substantial benefits from these methods. Self-directed teams can reduce costs and improve quality, the quality of work life, and productivity. Many of these companies report productivity improvements in the range of 30 to 50 percent when teams replace the old methods (Hoerr, Pollack, and Whiteside, 1986).

Reducing Levels of Management

Most healthcare and other organizations have more levels of management than they need or can use effectively. This has been the result of a slow process of change, for which there are several explanations. First, people have been promoted to management positions so that organizations could pay them enough money to retain them. Such promotions often result from compensation systems that use management responsibility as a key basis for salary level. Second, there has been a narrow span of control, in which some managers only have two to five people reporting to them. This leads to a "tall" organization. Third, responsibility and authority have not been delegated to the people performing the work. Consequently, all questions must be taken to one or more managers. If (as is often the case) a lower-level employee's recommendation is sound and ends up being followed, a substantial amount of time and money has been wasted.

One way to improve quality and reduce costs is to reduce the levels of management. Extra people in communication and decision-making cycles increase the time needed to reach a decision and increase the likelihood of information errors. The following recommendations are offered as approaches to reducing the levels of management:

1. Delegate responsibility and authority to the people performing the activities. Clearly, these people must be trained for their new responsibilities. They also need to understand the organizational and departmental mission and values, so that they will understand the context for their actions. They should be given some guidelines for the scope of their decisions (for example, "Settlements can be made up to a value of $1,000"). An information system will be required, to monitor their decisions. It is a good idea to delegate gradually, so that everyone gains experience and confidence. According to Kirby (1989, pp. 35–36), "Delegation is like any new skill; it takes time, persistence, and learning from mistakes. As you delegate, analyze what you did right and what could have been done better. As mistakes happen, keep people involved. Don't snatch the task away. Say those little words, 'Where do we go from here?' Eventually, everyone will get comfortable with the shared responsibility."

2. Pay staff the amounts required to retain them, on the basis of their contributions and competitive market salaries. Do not arbitrarily promote people just to pay them more. Use job expansion as a way to increase salaries. The more practical and difficult task is removing managerial titles from people who

have had them, even if they are paid the same salaries. This will be viewed as demotion.

3. Expect managers to have a relatively broad span of control after their employees have gained experience with delegated responsibility and authority. A broad span of control should be common. Professionals know their jobs and should require only broad guidance and coaching.

4. Use attrition as both a stimulus and a mechanism for reducing levels of management. When a manager leaves, the necessity for retaining the position should be evaluated. The organization can be changed at this time without terminating or demoting anyone.

5. Focus on process, rather than on the historical organizational structure. Combining functions within a process is an effective way of improving communication and working relationships. For example, preadmission review, admitting, and patient-account functions for inpatient services can be combined.

Work Reorganization and Reassignment

Another important component of reorganizing the way we work is work reorganization and reassignment. We must look carefully at the activities performed by people in each job category, to reassess knowledge and skill requirements. It may be possible to reorganize work and reassign selected activities to people in other job categories. Work reevaluation is most necessary in the professions that are most expensive and in shortest supply. In hospitals and nursing homes, registered nurses and allied health professionals fall into this category. Look at ways to provide assistance to these people.

It is best to maintain an open attitude about approaches to work reorganization and reassignment. Encourage managers, staff, customers, and suppliers to suggest new alternatives, and test those that offer the greatest opportunities for improvement. No single approach works in all circumstances.

One useful method is analysis of the activities, knowledge, and skills required in each position. Another approach is to focus on the activities involved throughout a process. With either approach, the first step is to develop a list of all activities and decisions. Next, you collect data on the frequency with which each activity and decision occurs over a sample time period and summarize the data. This summary provides information about the percentage distributions of activities and decisions. Next comes a careful analysis of each activity and decision, to determine the minimum level of knowledge and skill required. This part of the analysis is the most difficult because it challenges historical and current practices in work assignment, challenges perceptions of professional practice, and requires interpretations of abilities that are not currently being used. A multidisciplinary evaluation team should include the types of managers and professionals currently and potentially involved. Next, the potential work reassignments are combined with the frequency data, to evaluate the staffing impact of the reassignments. Finally, alternative configurations of work assignments should be tested in selected work areas or in portions of the overall process. The goals of the organization, department, or process should be translated into measures of quality and performance, to evaluate the success of the pilot tests. Successful alternatives can then be used more broadly.

We used this approach to analyze the work of registered nurses at the University of Michigan Hospitals, as part of a nursing activity study. The activities and decisions performed by nurses were listed for each inpatient care unit. The study was a group effort, involving the directors of nursing, head nurses, staff nurses, and management-systems consultants. Activities were grouped into categories of hygiene, nutrition, elimination, physical activity, safety, vital signs and monitoring, medications and IVs, special treatments/procedures, assessment, teaching, and emotional support, among others. Overall, we ended up with a set of activities applicable to all units, with additional activities unique to each unit. The frequency of each activity performed and required on each shift, for every inpatient on every unit, was documented over a sample period. The data were then summarized, and time standards were established for each activity. This process provided documentation, for each unit, of the time necessary (on the basis of current nursing practice) to perform all required activities. The next step was to carefully evaluate the knowledge and skills required for each of the activities and develop work-reassignment alternatives for pilot testing. This information is being used as a basis for planning staffing and reassignment of activities to staff members other than nurses.

Self-Directed Work Teams

Increasing numbers of organizations in the United States are moving to self-directed work teams as a way to revitalize and renew themselves.

Cultural Characteristics of Success. Many successful companies have adopted the principles of self-directed work teams. What made these companies opt for a change of such magnitude? There are some relevant characteristics in the cultures common to these corporations. First, they all have stated missions and goals and have worked to achieve broad understanding and shared aims and beliefs throughout the organization. Second, they know their customers, both internal and external, and frequently check requirements to make sure they are staying on track. Third, they know the competition well. They conduct frequent surveys and use "mystery shopper" techniques to maintain their knowledge base. Fourth, they believe in, and invest in, their employees through continuous training. Fifth, they support employees' empowerment and have given people sufficient freedom to function at the highest possible level. Sixth, the climate in these organizations is one of high expectation and high performance. Finally, the companies have flattened out the hierarchy, to allow employees to communicate effectively throughout the company. In essence, these companies have begun organizational transformation.

Before self-directed teams can begin, you must identify barriers to change, so that they can be dealt with early. Since self-directed teams function autonomously, certain conditions must be present before the organization can benefit from this work method. It must be possible to arrange tasks into a more meaningful whole by combining multiple skills, a high level of commitment and support from the top, and a group of personnel willing to experiment with a new organizational model.

In organizations with self-directed teams, management retains authority for the development of business objectives, overall work standards, codes of ethics, and definitions of the scope of work teams. The work teams plan, set priorities, organize, coordinate with others, measure, and take corrective action. All of these duties were previously the prerogative of management. Work teams solve problems, schedule and assign work, and handle such personnel issues as absenteeism. Team members also interview and hire new employees. Work teams encourage a climate for creativity and innovation and promote individual employees' becoming more involved. As Jack Richy, a general foreman at Bethlehem Steel, says, "The old style of management was adversarial. Now we are using people and their experience" (Labich, 1989).

Self-directed teams not only can accomplish the assigned work but also may be delegated many of the duties formerly handled by management. In essence, the self-directed team manages itself. On a self-directed team, the worker has broad responsibilities, not just a singular set of tasks. As workers learn new skills, they are in more broadly defined roles and can make increasing contributions. The goal is to allow each worker to experiment with different methods and ways of doing things, to bring creativity and innovation to work.

Traditionally, roles in healthcare organizations have been divided into many different categories, and there has been much specialization. Even a simple task, such as the transportation of patients to various ancillary departments, has been broken into specialized functions (separate transportation departments for radiology, physical therapy, nuclear medicine, and other areas). Jobs are so narrowly defined that employees have been kept from working outside their job descriptions. This has led to the phrase so many of us hate to hear: "It's not in my job description." The lack of a macro viewpoint, because of a hierarchical system of communication and the narrow definition of jobs, can

Table 4. Implementation Model for a Self-Directed Work Team.

Assess	Pilot	Implement	Integrate
Conduct a cultural audit	Share the vision	Begin the process	Select broad sites
Develop a feasibility study	Ask for volunteers	Monitor	Restructure rewards
Identify key leaders	Educate leaders and teams	Institutionalize	
Craft the vision	Build the teams		Evaluate

cause the feeling of alienation reported by so many American workers today.

As healthcare becomes more competitive and resources become more constrained, we need to find new, flexible ways of organizing that will help us broaden functions and organize for success. Consider how much more effective a centralized team of transporters with a singular dispatch center would be than several small units with narrow job definitions; one could take advantage of economies of scale and new technology to revamp the work to be done. Inviting workers to lend their expertise to the redesign will help you achieve their ownership of the process as they understand and learn to facilitate change.

Preparing to Implement Self-Directed Work Teams. If you feel that a more involved and productive work force can make a difference to your organization, you may wish to implement a self-directed work team. The team establishes its own work schedules and work flows, to meet requirements. The team analyzes its work flow and streamlines the process. Managers who have developed this minitransformation report lower staff turnover, higher staff morale, and higher productivity. Team members desire to be cross-trained for multiple functions. The model we suggest for implementation has been successfully used in financial services at the University of Michigan Hospitals. The model, illustrated in Table 4, has four steps: assess, pilot, implement, and integrate.

Action Step: **Assess or evaluate your organization. Consider conducting a cultural audit to assess the institution's readiness for change.**

During this process, you need to identify both formal and informal leaders. Remember to include managers, union leaders, and employee leaders. You will want to enlist these people as sponsors of your process.

Action Step: **Develop educational brainstorming sessions, where you can outline the vision, and ask these groups to review and edit your plans for reorganizing the way work is done. Make sure you have enlisted the support of top leaders before you go public with the plans, and review the conceptual framework of the process to make sure that it is compatible with overall organizational goals.**

Action Step: **Develop a feasibility study. Evaluate organizational readiness for streamlining, and develop an action plan. The plan will include the strategy for implementation and an evaluation process.**

As you consider various approaches, do not be restricted by resources. Envision the ideal first, and then backtrack mentally to design the right vision for your organization. The idea is to be as creative as possible. With key leaders of the organization, you should review the strategy for implementation and develop some key milestone dates, so that the process can be monitored. Then people will know what to expect.

Action Step: **Identify key formal and informal leaders and stakeholders in your organization and educate them.**

At the University of Michigan Hospitals, we set up a task force on work reorganization to steer the process and educate people about the concept. People throughout the organization with ideas for various projects used this task force as a steering group, to review proposals and develop team objectives. The task force also helped the first team develop ground rules and an evaluation model for the pilot.

In the second phase, a plan is developed to implement several pilot teams in a variety of departments across the organization. This is an effort to have the team model take root.

***Action Step*: Create a task force that can relate work reorganization to the mission, and attract volunteers to propose pilot projects in various areas of the organization.**

Training. Training for the process is a key ingredient of success. Managers should first be oriented to the concepts, and then they should participate in general orientation sessions with the teams. Training must be conducted with sensitivity, because managers and supervisors need to learn a whole new set of skills for this new work environment. The best of all possible worlds exists when a manager volunteers his or her area for a pilot test after hearing about the project outline; you know in advance that there is a level of readiness that will assist with implementation.

A planning retreat, to introduce the concepts of self-directed teams, should take place before implementation. Before the first retreat, however, it would be helpful for team members to have a chance to visit an organization where teams have been functioning. Alternatively, a seminar can offer an opportunity to hear from employees and a supervisor who have worked successfully with the team concept. This will help employees develop an understanding of what to expect. The curriculum for the retreat should include the following elements:

- Presentations on the benefits of self-directed work teams
- Discussion of why some teams work well and others fail

- An opportunity for teams to discuss their purposes and formulate goals
- Definitions of where the teams currently are in their development
- Definitions of where they would like to be
- Lists of barriers to successful implementation, to be developed by the teams in a working session
- Action plans to remove the barriers

Once the introduction has taken place, the team can discuss how to learn the new skills necessary to autonomous functioning.

Each team should have a facilitator, assigned in the beginning stages, to assist with training and trouble-shooting for the team. The facilitator can discuss how to learn such new skills as timekeeping, preparing budgets, assigning work, solving problems, training team members, setting team goals, resolving internal conflicts, and evaluating peer performance and team achievement. Such new concepts as flexible thinking must also be learned, and cross-functional training must occur. As you can see, the amount of required learning is extensive, and a heavy initial commitment to training is the only way to achieve strong teams.

We suggest that facilitators of different projects meet regularly, to share their successes and failures and handle questions about the process. Because facilitators are breaking new ground, they should keep notes on team development, to help in the training of future teams and facilitators. The development of teams takes a long time, but the payoff for the organization is great.

Management's Role. In the first phase of training, managers are encouraged to listen more effectively to workers' suggestions and discuss how they can be implemented. Managers also need to learn how to share information, keep workers informed, and provide encouragement and feedback.

Adequate preparation of managers for this change is essential. Time must be spent to develop seminars that teach the skills your managers will need. Sessions should be participatory, so that managers will feel comfortable expressing concerns about their new roles. An important way to lessen anxiety is to say that any reductions in management will be handled through attrition, rather than through layoffs. This statement makes it clear that the new philosophy will not eliminate jobs, and saying so may help you overcome resistance.

Changes in the Role of Supervisors. In an organization that sponsors self-directed teams, the role of the first-line supervisor becomes that of coach, mentor, and teacher. Rather than measuring and monitoring progress toward goals, the manager establishes the goals with team members and counsels them on goal achievement. This concept can be frightening to supervisors when it is first discussed, because of the radical change in responsibilities and duties. Fear may also result from the current tendency to reduce levels of management and first-line supervisors. Supervisors will have to recognize the newfound independence, learn to back away from tight control, and focus on helping the teams. In companies where teams have been installed, supervisors report renewed and enhanced job satisfaction. They also report feeling that they finally are helping their employees do their jobs better, rather than spending time disciplining people.

Responsibilities of Self-Directed Teams. The transition to self-directed teams requires a new way of thinking for employees. Every team member must play by the established guidelines and be responsible for his or her own work as a member of the team. Initiative must come from the individual instead of from the supervisor. Productivity and quality also become responsibilities of employees and their teams, rather than solely management's concerns. Skills necessary for team decision making must also be learned. Self-directed teams reward teamwork. Individual acquisition of skills allows for personal and professional growth. It is up to the members of the team to develop a self-learning schedule. The organization should facilitate this process by having appropriate tools available, such as computer-assisted learning aids, videotapes, and reading materials. Group facilitators and managers can also help anyone who may have a special learning problem.

Skill-development workshops will facilitate smooth transition. The major stumbling block to success in the transitional phase is that familiar behaviors are gone, and this loss of predictability can be frightening and counterproductive for employees and managers. The program must be tailored to support people as they become familiar with the new value system.

Discipline of employees who perform inadequately is commonly a shared responsibility of the team and management. Since teams participate in defining expectations for each team member, the teams can identify someone who does not perform to expectations. Teams apply a lot of group pressure on their members to perform as expected. Management must still work with the team leader to initiate appropriate additional training or disciplinary action.

> *Action Step*: **Provide as many opportunities for education, learning, and skill development as possible, both within your organization and in conjunction with local educational institutions. Arrange visits to corporations where teams have been functioning effectively.**

When teams have completed their generic training, the next step is to develop a clear understanding of the team's mission, role, and responsibilities. If the mission is not clear, it follows that nothing else will proceed well. Agreeing on a mission seems like a very simple step; nevertheless, having watched many a team try to define its mission and its relationship to the mission of the organization, we can tell you that it is not so easy. Team members may have never talked before about their raison d'être.

The next step in the process is to identify critical success factors and measures of performance. What will it take to succeed? A medical staff might agree, for example, to change the system for medical records. There should be a list of seven to ten factors that will become guidelines for the year. Once this organizational framework is in place, the team can proceed with learning the new skills and going repeatedly through the Plan-Do-Check-Act cycle. Performance must be measured regularly, to determine whether the changes have been successful.

Education and Participation of the Union. If there are unions in your organization, you must involve them early in the process. Early meetings with union leaders to explain goals, process steps, and benefits may help you avoid the kind of failure that is due to lack of communication. In most cases, unions support work reorganization, as long as they can participate in and understand the changes.

Union members have certain common concerns:

1. *Involvement in decisions:* This is particularly an issue for unions in such professions as nursing. Several approaches to allowing greater involvement and authority for employees have been discussed in this chapter.
2. *Job security:* This is an issue particularly when an organization has implemented or faces cost reductions. You cannot gain a union's support if its members will be terminated. Attrition should be used as the primary approach to reducing staff.
3. *Salaries, benefits, and rewards:* Unless specifically negotiated otherwise, union contracts tend to base salaries on job classifications and years of service, not on contributions to the performance of the organization.

Action Step: **Restructure the reward system to favor team development and progress, rather than individual progress and achievement.**

Team rewards based on performance of the group or organization as a whole are normally acceptable to unions because they are also in the best interests of employees.

Identification of Barriers. There are many barriers to successful implementation of self-directed work teams, such as lack of top management's support, lack of the union's support, an environment where failures are punished, inadequate resources, threatened first-line or middle managers, inability to deal with existing institutional boundaries, inappropriate levels of control, inability of teams to make decisions, and poor communication with other parts of the organization that are not part of the pilot effort. The key to success is identifying and removing the barriers. Your survey of the institution should list any barriers that may interfere with teams' progress. Teams should work on developing action plans to remove these barriers before the implementation phase.

Corporate Commitment. Commitment from the top is as critical in this process as it is in any other major organizational change. Employees must see sincere commitment from the top before they will be willing to invest in a new work method. There have been many false starts in trying to turn organizations around. If top leaders do not become actively involved, an effort looks like just another program to the workers. There tends to be a built-in inertia in these cases, and workers are content to develop a "wait and see" attitude.

Many companies have been successful in piloting a few demonstration units, in which self-directed teams can be tested and success can be highlighted for the rest of the organization.

Action Step: **Be visible and enthusiastic in supporting the team concept.**

Summary

A more involved work force is valuable for many reasons. Committed employees are effective in reducing costs, improving quality, creating a more rewarding work life, and enhancing job satisfaction. Many organizations that have converted to team concepts and use the most radical innovation — semiautonomous work teams — are far more successful than their conventional counterparts.

The organizational culture must be changed to allow risk

taking. The goal should be encouraging people to learn from their mistakes, rather than punishing them for errors. It is essential to plan and benefit from a diverse multicultural environment.

Whether you choose employee involvement or self-directed work teams, the principle is to allow employees to enhance the organization while developing their personal abilities and skills. In these participative models, everyone can be a winner.

> *Action Step*: **Develop a climate where risk taking is rewarded and mistakes are viewed as opportunities for learning.**

Chapter Nine

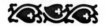

Promoting Success
as Everyone's Role

What Is Success?

To promote the concept that everyone must play a role in achieving organizational success, we must first define *success*. In its simplest form, success is high achievement (according to the measures of success used). For your organization, success can be judged by several measures. Probably the most important measure of success for an organization is its continued existence. Hospitals, nursing homes, and other organizations that have been in business for many years are generally judged successful. Common measures of organizational success are (1) the ability to meet the organization's goals, such as continued existence, education, or care for a specific population; (2) community service; and (3) profitability, particularly when owners have purchased the organization for the express purpose of making a profit, rather than for some other purpose, such as providing quality products or services (entrepreneurs tend to have a passion for a particular product or service, while later investors often do not).

The success of an organization usually depends on many people. For a healthcare organization, physicians, board members, nurses, therapists, suppliers, and others can contribute to overall success.

Personal success can also be judged via several measures, but these are normally different from those used for the organization. Personal success is judged by such measures as income, education, recognition, meeting of personal goals, and enjoyment. It is important to realize that although some measures of

172

success are similar, every employee has different personal goals. Two people working as aides in a nursing home may have very different personal objectives. One may be working to support a family, so that money, fringe benefits, and availability of over-time work may be very important. Another person may be a supplemental wage earner, working primarily for the enjoyment of helping patients. For such a person, money and fringe benefits may be secondary. In all cases, people want to avoid environments where personal success is in conflict with organizational success.

The key to involving everyone in success is to develop complementary measures of business and personal success. To maximize success, you must develop a win-win situation with everyone involved. Leaders and managers must recognize the interdependence of organizational and personal success.

Points of Decision

With an effort of an individual or a single-person company, there is a single point of decision. The person understands all known information, understands the common goals and objectives, and participates in any gains or losses. There is no inherent conflict between goals and measures of success.

This does not mean, however, that the individual has complete knowledge, nor does it mean that he or she does not have to make trade-offs among goals. We all know that, because of limited resources, we cannot meet every desired goal in our personal or business life. Moreover, individual priorities and decisions also change, as goals change over time and as additional information becomes available. At the time of a decision, however, there is no conflict of opinion.

With a multiperson organization, however, goals, information, and decisions are very dispersed. Each person has a partial and different understanding of information. There are also differing personal goals, different concepts of organizational goals and objectives, and differing levels of participation in financial gain and loss. The larger the company, the wider the dispersion. This dispersion leads to conflicting decisions and suboptimization of success. The issues are the degree of suboptimization and who experiences it.

As a simple example, consider a two-person practice in orthopedic surgery. One surgeon has been in the practice for fifteen years, and the second surgeon joined last year. Now consider two alternative scenarios for business and personal success. In the first scenario, the senior surgeon attends professional meetings in the most exclusive and expensive locations, takes 70 percent of the practice's net income, and rarely works nights, weekends, or holidays. As long as money is coming in, the senior surgeon has high individual success. But the junior surgeon is proportionately overworked, underpaid, and disgruntled. The success measures of the business and the two surgeons are incompatible. The junior surgeon will tend to avoid new cases, minimize time with patients (to their dissatisfaction), and begin looking for a new position. In this case, the success of the practice suffers, since it is losing business, losing customers' satisfaction, and will lose a surgeon. The second scenario involves a more equitable distribution of professional meetings, work, and income. In this case, the junior surgeon aggressively works to build an enduring and expanding practice. Business success is improved, and combined individual success is also improved. The senior surgeon's individual short-term success is diminished, but her long-term business and personal success will be improved. The key is sharing and cooperation.

To reduce the discrepancies among organizational and personal success, you must disperse information more effectively and find ways to share benefits and losses with the people involved. This will build ownership, which is the key to mutual organizational and individual success, as discussed later in this chapter.

Overcoming Barriers to Success

There are many barriers to everyone's seeing organizational success as part of his or her role.

Lack of Common Goals. Probably the single most important barrier to organizational success is the lack of common mission, vision, values, and goals, or the lack of integrated goals.

Differences Between Management's and Staff's Benefits. Most organizations provide their managers perquisites (perks) not available to other employees. The issue is the degree of difference in rewards. Very few employees will argue that managers should not have higher pay, nicer offices, and better benefits. When management enjoys what are perceived as excessively different perks, however, employees become resentful. They see business success and their personal success as jeopardized by the individual success of managers. For example, consider the multimillion-dollar compensation packages of top executives in the U.S. automobile industry. Only recently have some U.S. automobile company employees been eligible for bonuses based on the success of the business. We are familiar with many auto company managers and employees at Ford Motor Company. To judge from our personal sample, the attitudes of these employees are now more focused on Ford's organizational success because they see it as tied to their individual success.

Action Step: **Consider restructuring the reward system for employees, with greater emphasis on group improvements and fewer evaluation categories for individuals.**

Lack of Commitment to Employees. Employees will not be committed to the organization unless they perceive that the organization has some commitment to them.

Management's Separation from Day-to-Day Activities. Many managers, especially top executives, have become separated from the day-to-day activities of the organization. Managers spend the large majority of their time involved in meetings within their own areas, and they miss opportunities to see and communicate with employees. For example, the CEO of a large hospital had an appointment with the chief of pathology. For

some reason, the CEO had scheduled the meeting in the pathologist's office, but the pathologist's office was no longer in its
former location; it had moved over five years earlier. The CEO's
arrival at the former location, now a laboratory, alarmed a
laboratory worker, who thought that she was certainly in trouble
because the CEO was there. This anecdote simply illustrates how
rarely the CEO visited operational areas.

*Competition Among Professional Groups and Organiza-
tional Departments.* Competition has become a way of life for
Americans. From the time we start school, cooperation is considered cheating; in fact, cooperation among large corporations
is illegal. Yet competition is often counter-productive. In many
situations, cooperation produces a better outcome for everyone,
particularly within an organization.

Most healthcare organizations experience competition
among professional groups and among departments. Nurses
and pharmacists compete for management and administration
of drugs. Departments commonly conduct turf wars involving
functions, employees, and budgets. Each department attempts
to optimize its own objectives at someone else's expense.

Lack of Support for Learning. Most organizations inadvertently discourage continued learning. Other than in the clinical
professions, there are few expectations for employees in
healthcare organizations to continue their learning. For example, what types of continuing education and training are provided for receptionists? Most organizations restrict tuition reimbursement to work-related courses, if they reimburse tuition at
all.

Action Step: **Identify the barriers that exist in your
organization, and work to reduce them.**

It is important for you to identify barriers to success and
continual improvement. Set priorities and select one or more
for immediate attention.

Cautions and Environmental Considerations

Leaders should promote innovation and change, but some cautions are in order.

Change Takes Time. We have all learned our beliefs, attitudes, and actions over many years, and we have often learned behavior informally. It will take several years to fully change behavior and the corporate culture. Physicians, employees, and others will respond to actions that exhibit the new philosophies more than they will respond to written or spoken statements. Most managers and staff people believe that talk is cheap; they want to see real action.

Bad Decisions Outweigh Good Decisions. Managers' decisions and actions that are inconsistent with the new goals will be noticed more quickly and more widely than decisions and actions that are consistent. The consequences of inconsistent and bad actions have approximately five times the impact of consistent and good actions.

Actions to Promote Success as Everyone's Role

Chapter Four discussed revitalizing the mission and values of your organization. If you want everyone in your organization to promote and contribute to its success, then organizational goals must be compatible with the goals of all the people involved.

There should be a hierarchy of goals for the organization as a whole, for major divisions, for departments, and for individuals. All of these goals must be consistent with the organization's values, which means difficult decisions about priorities, roles, and sharing gains and losses.

Action Step: **Establish compatible organizational and individual goals.**

Basic to promoting success is communicating with *every* person involved in any way with your organization. You cannot expect people to promote success for your organization if they are uninformed or if the organization's measures of success are incompatible with their personal measures of success. Every individual must be able to see his or her role in the context of the mission, values, and goals of the department, division, and organization.

Give copies of mission, values, and goals statements to every current and new board member, physician, employee, and supplier. These are your partners in accomplishing organizational success. Provide descriptions or excerpts regularly in written communications, such as newsletters, letters to employees, and posters. People must be informed before they can be expected to promote your organization's success.

Action Step: **Communicate with everyone involved.**

People and teams who know and demonstrate the values and goals of the organization should be rewarded, but not necessarily with money. Recognition alone is a powerful motivator. One approach is for senior managers to stop people in the halls and ask them about the organization's values or goals. If people know the values, compliment them or give them a free meal in the cafeteria. NKC, Inc. (Louisville, Kentucky), has used this approach and even created a form of internal money called "quality bucks," which are redeemable at the cafeteria and the gift shop. Another approach is to identify people who demonstrate the desired actions and reward them. The University of Michigan Hospitals use a "mystery guest" to identify people who are particularly helpful to patients and other guests at the hospitals. These helpful people are then recognized in an internal publication.

Action Step: **Recognize those who demonstrate knowledge of the values and goals.**

What are the goals of your board members, physicians, employees, and suppliers? This information is particularly important for the people who will be leading your organization. It also contributes to employee development, rewards, and recognition. General (anonymous) surveys are useful for determining the compatibility between organizational and individual goals (this information is helpful in evaluating the organization's goals), overall opinions about common programs, and potential options for rewards and recognition.

A good approach to improving compatibility between organizational and individual success is to survey opinions as organizational goals are being established or revised and as people are assigned to different roles. For example, if a person basically does not like disabled, elderly patients, that person is incompatible with the goals of a nursing home, even if he or she is willing to take the job for the salary. The attitudes and goals of potential medical staff members, employees, and suppliers should be measured before you establish any relationship with them, to the extent that such measurement is practical and legal. If there are significant incompatibilities, for example, between an applicant and a particular position, the person should be considered for another position. Every manager should seek employees and suppliers who genuinely like the business.

Action Step: Solicit information on personal goals.

NKC, Inc., has developed a useful way of looking at this relationship: it is called *ownership*. Although employees are not actually owners of the organization, NKC wants them to share the organization's values and act to achieve success for the organization. If we want employees to act as owners, we must treat them as owners. We recommend the following approaches used at NKC (Stansbury, 1989):

1. *Provide employees with ownership information.* Offer complete information about how the department and the organization are doing. Tell employees about customers' feedback and planned changes. Keep employees informed. Communicate with them.

2. *Support innovation and risk taking.* Customers' requirements should be communicated (see Chapter Five). Then em-

ployees should be encouraged, in many ways, to understand and meet them. At NKC, all employees are expected to help people who need help and, if necessary, personally escort them to their destinations. It is acceptable for employees to be away from their normal work stations to help customers. This is the way an owner would act; we should also allow our employees to act this way.

3. *Recognize and reward improvement efforts.* If you were an owner, you would be rewarded in some manner for improvements, if only by positive feedback from customers.

4. *Remove barriers to quality improvement.* As an owner, you want to remove any barriers to providing better products and services to your customers.

Suppliers, by working closely with your organization, can meet your internal requirements and the requirements of your customers. Suppliers understand their services and products better than anyone else does and are in a position to improve performance, if you treat them as partners.

> *Action Step:* **Treat physicians, employees, and suppliers as partners.**

Your organization should clearly express its expectation of commitment from employees, as well as its commitment to them. If employees have no sense of security or commitment from the organization, they will not invest any personal time or energy. They will focus on money and short-term objectives because they will have no trust in the future. Professional athletes illustrate this point perfectly. A professional football player knows very well that the team will fire him whenever a better player is found, if his performance is not up to expectations, if he is injured, or if for some other reason he falls out of favor. Consequently, the athlete negotiates for the absolute maximum salary and benefits that he can get in the short term; some are now negotiating multiyear-term contracts.

Employees want job security, but it is unrealistic to guarantee jobs. In today's risky, competitive environment, it is very difficult for organizations to assure employees of a long-term future. The new corporate takeovers have also complicated commitments for the future. Nevertheless, you can do some things to demonstrate commitment:

1. Make employee reductions through attrition. Improved productivity in healthcare organizations will usually mean fewer employees. Some will retire, move, or leave for other reasons. In general, attrition will run at least 4 to 10 percent per year. This means that planned staff reductions of 4 to 10 percent per year can be accomplished without current employees losing their jobs. In large organizations, the attrition rate is relatively stable, but in small organizations it may not be so predictable. Since there are limits to retraining, there are limits to filling positions with internal candidates. For example, without several years of education, a housekeeper cannot be retrained as a registered nurse, but a housekeeper can be trained as a pharmacy or dietetics aide. An organization should attempt to fill positions with existing personnel whenever possible.

2. Identify poorly performing employees, and provide training and counseling to help them improve. Most employees will respond to this assistance; if not, they should be transferred to other positions or terminated. Employees who perform poorly are recognized by their peers and can ruin the morale and motivation of other employees.

3. Provide training, retraining, and education for employees. The employees will recognize the investment in them.

4. Offer attractive exit packages. Early retirement, lump-sum exit payments, and other options have been used successfully to induce employees to leave and pursue other options.

5. Help employees find positions elsewhere. If reductions must be made, cover employees financially during the transition and help them find new positions that they are happy with, and your remaining employees will not feel threatened.

Action Step: **Establish two-way commitment.**

Healthcare leaders and managers should become visibly involved in two-way communications with physicians, managers, employees, suppliers, and customers. Two-way communication builds both understanding and the trust necessary for promoting the mutual success of the organization and individuals. Here are some suggestions:

1. Meet with employees in open forums. The chief executive officer, chief operating officer, or chief of the medical staff should participate in open employee meetings.
2. When wandering around, talk to employees at all levels. Ask about something specific; don't just say hello.
3. Provide several mechanisms for every employee to receive and provide information.
4. Make regular rounds of all facilities. Sam Walton, chairman of Wal-Mart, still personally attends the opening of every store (there are now over seven hundred); employees know he cares (Peters and Austin, 1985).
5. Hold meetings in departments or work areas, rather than in executive offices. You will accomplish two objectives. First, you will learn by visiting many areas of your organization. Second, people in those areas will know that you have seen their situation.
6. Establish an employee suggestion program, to provide a good mechanism for employees' communications.

Action Step: **Become visibly involved in two-way communication.**

As we have said, visualization is a powerful tool. The ability to mentally remove yourself from your current situation and imagine a situation from many perspectives can help you become more creative. First, view the situation overall. No matter which side of an issue you are on, ask what is best for customers and what is best for the organization. Second, view the situation from the perspective of other people. Imagine yourself as an employee, a patient, or someone else in the situation. What would you be concerned about? The ability to visualize is easy to develop. This is a very powerful way to improve decision making. This approach improves compatibility between organizational and individual goals.

> *Action Step*: **Visualize yourself in other people's situations.**

Trust must be earned. With any change, the best way to earn trust is to make your decisions and actions consistent with your statements. To build trust, leaders and managers must demonstrate and communicate actions consistent with the organization's values. You must say what you mean and mean what you say.

> *Action Step*: **Establish trust.**

Innovation and creativity were discussed in Chapter Seven. One approach to encouraging employees to promote the success of the organization is to establish formal programs that solicit, recognize, and reward new ideas and innovations. The programs should address at least three different forms of contribution, as follow.

Cost Reduction. These programs are the easiest to justify because any funds for rewards and implementation can be paid out of savings. Analysis of and rewards for these programs should address the time and marginal impacts of a cost reduction. For example, a program may recognize first-year cost reductions only. Will savings include *any* calculated reductions, or only items that can be demonstrated as actual savings from the budget? For example, suppose that an average of one minute per bill is saved by a business office in a hospital or industrial corporation. That savings could be calculated as the average salary rate, times the number of bills, times the minute per bill. Alternatively, the savings could be calculated only as the payroll reduction for billers eliminated from the business office.

Revenue Increases. With these contributions, it is important to distinguish between gross revenue and net income. A customary definition of *revenue*, for most healthcare providers, is the sum of all charges, yet few payers pay full charges. Hence, the true benefit of changes or innovations that increase revenues should be calculated as the net of any allowances, bad debt, and other deductions. Calculate the bottom-line change in income to the organization. Two other distinctions are important for the calculations. First, are net incomes to be calculated for the first year only, for several years, or for the present value of all future years? Second, will price increases be allowed? Given that healthcare costs are considered excessive by most businesses and patients, some suggestion and innovation programs do not allow price increases as an approach to increasing revenue.

Quality Improvements in Services and Products. These are the most difficult programs to address with any quantitative rewards. Improvements in quality seldom have short-term identifiable financial impacts, although in the long run they may have major impacts on quality, market share, and longevity of the organization. One approach is to provide either greater recognition or minimal financial rewards. The risk is that there is a larger short-term benefit for employees in suggesting cost reductions and revenue increases than in suggesting quality improvements.

Action Step: **Establish an employee suggestion and/or innovation program.**

Two types of time frames and developmental efforts must also be distinguished. The first concerns changes that are immediately calculable and implementable or can be demonstrated and implemented within a few months. An example is a suggestion to install rubber bumpers on the edges of carts, to reduce the costs of repairing wall damage. The second concerns changes that require substantial time and investment to demonstrate and implement. An example would be a new product: a prototype must be developed, patents must be requested, production capacity must be located, marketing and sales outlets must be established, and so on. This could take two years or longer, and no one can project the final market impact or profitability. These innovations must be handled differently from those with demonstrable short-term benefits. One approach is to provide the innovator, or intrapreneur, with a percentage ownership of any benefits.

To promote success as everyone's role, leaders must remove barriers to success. One useful approach is to establish one or more processes to identify perceived barriers. Although it is possible to identify individuals responsible for perceived barriers, it is normally more productive to allow anonymity. Here are two possible approaches:

1. Request customers and suppliers to identify perceived barriers to any proposed change. These can then be prioritized and addressed.
2. Administer a structured analysis of current resistance to change among customers and suppliers. One example is the *Change Resistance Scale* (O.D. Resources, Inc., 1988).

   Action Step: **Establish a process for identifying barriers to success.**

Flexibility is important in recognizing the contributions of individuals. Since each person's goals and measures of success differ, a menu of choices should be provided:

- Money (this is mentioned first because most people think of it first, not because it is best)
- Broadened work assignments
- Special assignments in areas of special interest to individuals
- Business trips
- Assistance in preparing professional papers or presentations
- Flexible work hours
- Tuition reimbursement

- Time off or rescheduled work, to allow people to learn something new

There are many choices; but again, flexibility is the key. Ask people what they would like.

Action Step: Develop flexible systems for rewards and recognition.

Voluntary cooperation is based on some mutual benefit, or on sharing of good and bad outcomes. This is true for relationships among organizations and their departments, employees, and suppliers. Consider patient-transportation workers employed in more than one department. Each department is concerned about the availability of transportation, but cooperation makes fewer transporters necessary when all departments draw from a central pool.

Action Step: Share good and bad outcomes.

Revise Human Resources Systems

Many of the options available to managers for recognizing employees require no changes in personnel systems. For example, it costs nothing to recognize an employee among peers or in group meetings. Temporary changes in work assignments or job responsibility do not require revisions of the personnel system; you can be creative and ask for ideas from the people involved.

Nevertheless, some forms of reward and recognition are affected by human resources systems. Methods of hiring, evaluating, and compensating people have been developed to promote equity among employees with similar abilities, experience, and performance. Unfortunately, however, many human resources systems have become quite rigid. The challenge is to achieve reasonable equity among employees while still allowing flexibility of rewards and recognition.

One approach to achieving flexibility has been the "cafeteria" or "menu" benefits package. This arrangement allows employees to select different combinations of health insurance, life insurance, and so on. The same approach could be used to provide more flexibility in rewards and recognition. An employee or a department could be given a choice: time for research or education, an "expense account" to test an improvement, a temporary reassignment, and so on.

Action Step: **Develop a flexible human resources system.**

The degree of improvement your organization achieves will be related to the number of employees who contribute. Therefore, you must involve as many employees as you can.

Chapter Ten

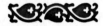

Improving
Cost-Effectiveness

Many changes in the healthcare industry are financial in nature and require organizations to become more cost-effective. This is especially true for healthcare providers. Unless healthcare providers become more cost-effective, they will encounter financial difficulties and their survival will be in jeopardy.

Most healthcare organizations have been undertaking cost-reduction programs for several years, with poor results. It is critical to distinguish cost-effectiveness from cost reduction. This chapter presents some ideas for improving cost-effectiveness. *Improving both quality and cost-effectiveness must be a continual effort based on system and process improvements.*

Terms and Concepts

Cost-effectiveness has two obvious components, cost and effectiveness, and is the ratio of cost to a level of effectiveness, which is a measure of value. To be successful, you must address the effectiveness issues first.

Effectiveness is "the degree or extent of achievement of objectives without regard for resource consumption" (Smalley, 1982, pp. 17–18). It is a measurement of how well the values, mission, and goals of your organization are being fulfilled. These must be established first and must be based on patients and other customers.

Cost reduction is simply the lowering of expenses, with no requirement that it address organizational priorities. Most cost-reduction programs have stated or unstated assumptions about the scope of services and products that will be retained. Unfortu-

188

nately, many assume that all services and products will be retained and equally penalized by across-the-board budget reductions. Organizations that jump immediately to across-the-board cost reductions face tremendous long-term risks because they have not determined their customers, requirements, and priorities. There is an assumption that the current stated and unstated objectives are correct, and that costs of meeting those objectives can simply be reduced, with no modification in the scope of products and services.

Efficiency is the dimensionless ratio of results or outputs, divided by the same measurements of inputs, expressed as a decimal or a percentage (Smalley, 1982). Efficiency is essentially the same thing as productivity except that outputs and inputs must be expressed in the same units of measurement. The goal of efficiency measurement is to minimize the resources needed to produce a given service or product.

Quality, as previously defined, has several different interpretations, probably the most useful of which involves meeting the customer's valid requirements.

Measurements of efficiency ignore the necessity for the service or product and the question of whether the service or product meets the customer's requirements. Cost-effectiveness addresses the dimensions of effectiveness and quality in meeting the customer's requirements, as well as resource cost to achieve that outcome.

An Approach to Improving Cost-Effectiveness

This section describes an approach to improving cost-effectiveness and quality in your organization. A process of twenty action steps is illustrated in Figure 21. This process should be a regular part of continual improvement. The initial steps coincide with the quality-improvement process discussed in Chapter Five. The steps discussed in this chapter describe additional actions to improve cost-effectiveness. The steps are illustrated in a logical sequence but may be performed in other sequences, according to what the situation requires. The initial steps described in Chapter Five are important in ensuring that

Figure 21. Action Steps to Improve Cost-Effectiveness.

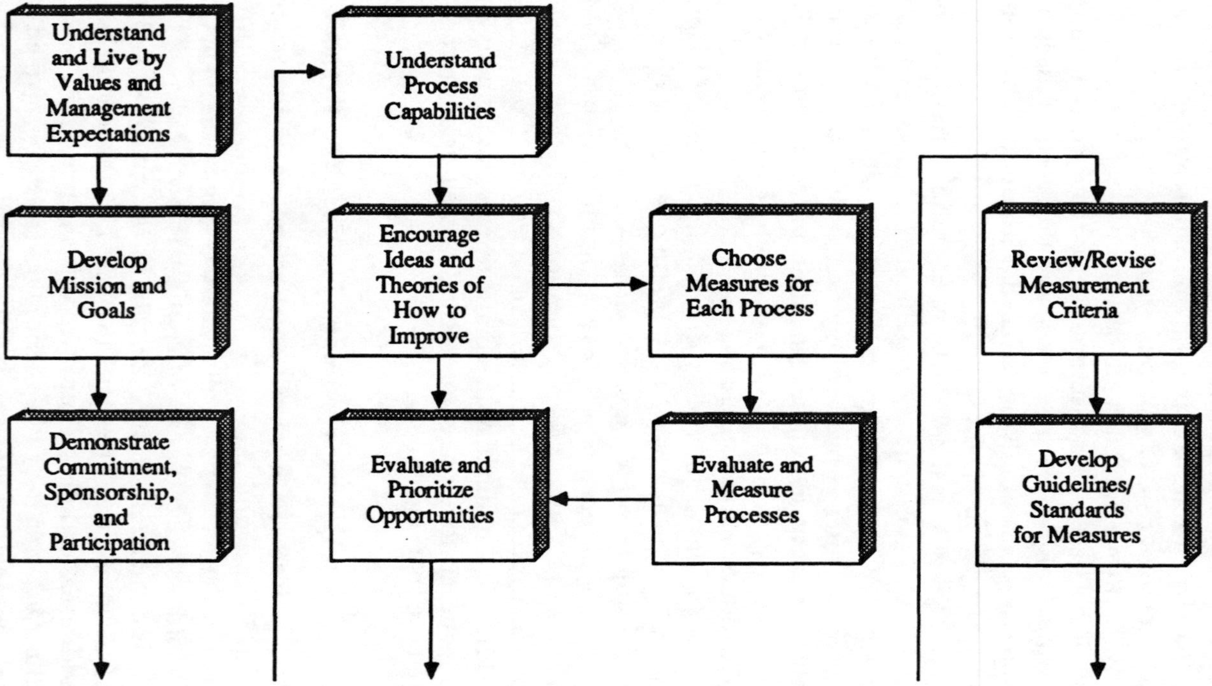

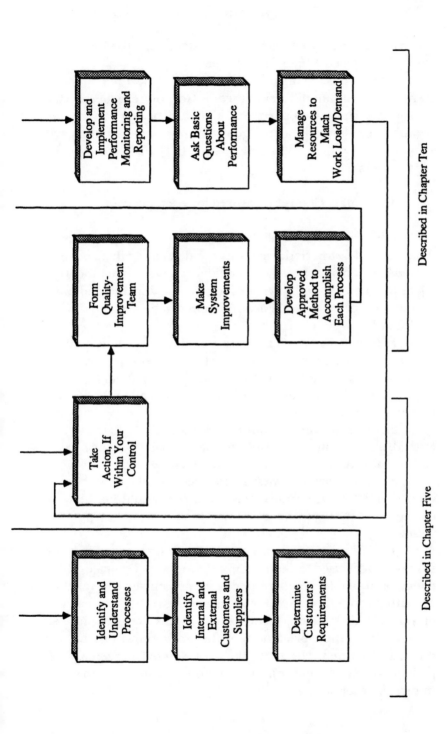

Described in Chapter Five

Described in Chapter Ten

Identify and Understand Processes

Identify Internal and External Customers and Suppliers

Determine Customers' Requirements

Take Action, If Within Your Control

Form Quality-Improvement Team

Make System Improvements

Develop Approved Method to Accomplish Each Process

Develop and Implement Performance Monitoring and Reporting

Ask Basic Questions About Performance

Manage Resources to Match Work Load/Demand

performance measurements are consistent with the organization's goals and customers' requirements.

The actions of corporate leaders and departmental managers are similar but different in scope. Corporate leaders focus on coordinating all departments and functions to meet the organizational mission and goals. Departmental managers focus on making process improvements that concern their departments.

Action Step: **Choose measures for each process.**

While it is not feasible to measure everything, there should be at least periodic measures to determine that customers' requirements are being met and that processes are functioning as planned. Quantitative progress can be documented only by measures of processes. Each function can be measured with the following types of criteria:

1. *Output measures*: These are measures of volume, quality, or service level. In most cases, customers' requirements are characteristics of the outputs (for example, a patient's getting well, total time the patient spent at the outpatient clinic, or cost of medications).

2. *Input measures*: Examples here include staff hours worked, quantity and quality of supplies used for a surgical case, and cost for meals in a long-term-care facility.

3. *Productivity measures*: These are ratios of output measures divided by input measures. Examples would be the cost per meal served, or the number of nursing hours per inpatient day.

4. *Utilization measures*: These are the percentages of available resources used. Examples would be the percentage occupancy of available inpatient beds, the percentage of available operating-room time used for surgical cases, or the percentage of available time during which exam rooms are occupied by patients. The appropriateness of the utilization must be addressed separately. For example, a substantial percentage of patients' time in exam rooms is commonly spent in waiting, not in receiving service.

5. *Financial and budget measures*: These are probably easiest to understand. Financial measures are very important. If an organization does not remain financially viable, it will cease to provide any services or products. One opportunity for improvement lies in converting to variable budgeting of staff, supplies, money, and other resources, according to the volume of services and products provided each month.

Before performance measures are implemented, they should be checked for appropriateness and consistency with the goals and objectives of the function, department, and organization where they will be used. It is particularly important that one department not optimize measurements that are detrimental to other departments or to the organization as a whole. This is a common problem when an organization's goals and total costs are not considered as part of the performance-measure establishment process. Individual managers, physicians, employees, and suppliers then optimize their own respective measures of performance, to the detriment of the organization as a whole. Ask these questions in verifying appropriateness: Does the measure support the organization's goals? What is its impact on the total costs, total revenues, and total profitability of the organization? Is the measure at the right level of emphasis? Is the measure useful for decisions? Is this measurement excessive? Is there a potential for misuse — beating the system by using the measure?

Action Step: **Evaluate and measure processes.**

The next step is to measure performance and evaluate the potential for improvement. Measurements should be graphed over time, to focus attention on the correct questions and the opportunities for change.

Several methods can be used to evaluate processes. These processes are described in many books on statistics and quality control. The objective is to ask the correct questions about special causes of variation versus common causes of variation. The purpose here is not to explain statistical methods but to indicate their usefulness in improving cost-effectiveness.

Action Step: **Form a quality-improvement team.**

A quality- or process-improvement team is appropriate to examining a process and developing improvements. You may have teams that work solely within single departments, but teams commonly include people from several departments. The team should be composed of vertical and horizontal cross-sections of managers and staff people working on the process, customers, and suppliers. Managers alone cannot effectively address problems or opportunities because they do not understand processes in detail. For example, a team formed to improve mail service might include responsible line managers, mail carriers, customers of the mail service, and possibly suppliers. Avoid teams larger than ten or twelve people unless the work can be divided. Input can be secured from others who are not on the working team. It is helpful to use a facilitator who is familiar with group dynamics, organizational change, and process-improvement techniques. The members of the team should be trained and coached in the scientific method, flow charting, statistical variation, process control, and other techniques.

As we have already pointed out, approximately 85 percent of performance improvements result from process changes implemented by staff members and customers. Most of these improvements flow from enhanced communications, which lead to enlightened, integrated management decisions. Decision-support systems provide leaders and managers with more complete and more timely information. According to Coffey, Gialanella, and Gilbert (1989, p. 5), decision-support systems "are generally defined as multidisciplinary combinations of people, resources, and information" that promote managers' decision making and "actively facilitate change." Effective decision-support systems "must address the full range of decisions facing senior and middle management, and integrate information and experience from multiple sources to achieve cost-effective and relevant decisions and actions." Improved cost-effectiveness depends heavily on managing quantitative and qualitative information about your processes.

Action Step: **Make system improvements.**

System or process improvements are one key to improved quality and cost-effectiveness and should be accomplished before any so-called standards are considered. A number of approaches are useful in identifying potential system improvements.

Prepare a flow chart of the current process. This is simply a picture of actions, movements, and decisions. Determine that value is added at each step of the flow chart. If it is not, try to eliminate that step. For example, if bills are simply moved from one location to another several times, no value is added toward the objective of mailing the bill to the payer. Any extra movement should be eliminated, so that quality will be improved and cost will simultaneously be reduced.

Ask a series of questions about the need and appropriate locations for activities. The purpose of the questions is to understand what is required and why. Is the activity required by law? If so, what are the minimum legal requirements? Is the activity required by an accreditation board or other professional organization? If so, what are the minimum requirements? Is the activity required by reimbursement organizations, such as Medicare, Medicaid, Blue Cross, or commercial insurance companies? If so, what are the minimum requirements? Is the activity required by organizational policy? If so, what are the minimum requirements? Is the activity required by the customers? If so, what are their requirements? Can the activity be eliminated? If you can avoid an activity, you eliminate all its costs.

Determine whether all the outputs of the process are required. For example, it is common for reports to be filled even when their contents are no longer relevant.

Can the activity be performed less frequently? One large hospital reevaluated the frequency with which rooms were cleaned. It was determined that offices and other low-traffic spaces were being cleaned far more frequently than they needed to be. The result was a 20 percent reduction in staffing, with no change in employee productivity.

Can the activity be done in a simpler, faster, easier, or more cost-effective manner? Instead of completing similar information on two forms, use one form with a carbon copy.

Can lower-skilled staff perform the activity? Using the right skill mix is a very important approach to reducing costs while still providing services and products. This is especially true with registered nurses and other healthcare professionals currently in short supply.

Can fewer or less expensive supplies be used? What are the inventories of bills, supplies, and other materials? Large inventories lead to high carrying costs, which result from delayed billing and unnecessary inventories.

Are services and products appropriately billed? Lost or inaccurate charges are common problems among healthcare organizations.

Downsizing

The need for and value of the current organizational structure should be challenged. Because healthcare organizations have been in a growth phase, many line, management, and overhead positions have been added. Success has meant growth, and big tends to breed bigger. The more successful an organization has been, the more likely it is to have added jobs and layers of management. The problem is that large organizations tend to be risk-averse, unimaginative, and ineffective. In most large organizations, people spend more energy justifying their territories and existence than improving processes and cost effectiveness. American business has recognized this tendency and is downsizing. According to Drucker (1988), in ten years the typical American business will have half the levels of management of its counterparts today and no more than one-third the number of managers.

Many industries are currently eliminating one or more levels of management hierarchy and broadening the span of control (see Figure 22). This approach, if properly implemented, is an effective way to improve productivity and cost-effectiveness. The current management literature proposes an increase in the numbers of people supervised by managers; but many organizations that have downsized have left their remaining supervisors overburdened, without appropriate training and skills. Such an approach to downsizing frequently creates frustration, mistrust, and low employee morale, and it does not improve productivity. Downsizing is effective only if the remaining people in the organization can assume the tasks once performed by the previous managers. This often becomes a test of managers' willingness to delegate authority and responsibility to employees lower in the organization, as well as their willingness to train those employees to perform their new roles successfully. In the downsizing of a healthcare organization, the following lessons should be considered (Tomasko, 1987; Solovy, 1988a).

1. Start before you have to. Planning is more effective if you are not under duress and have the time and resources to consider "what if" strategies, without the pressures of territorial protection.

2. Prepare for problems; think ahead. What are the possible problems, and what actions might you take? Think about the "80/20 rule." It is common for 80 percent of the impact to come from 20 percent of the activities. This rule allows you to focus on functions that will have the largest impact.

3. Use a rifle, not a shotgun. Focus on specific changes and implement them, rather than attempting everything at one time.

4. Continually manage size and shape. Any increases in size should be carefully scrutinized. Look at reallocation of resources. Practice thinking "lean and efficient." Do not fall into the trap of restoring positions when the pressure is off. This concept was named the "doom loop" by Philip Lathrop, a consultant who found that hospitals often restored jobs when the pressure was off (Solovy, 1988a).

5. Go after more than costs and jobs. Focus on process improvement instead. Process improvement leads to improved quality and cost-effectiveness. Keep the focus on organizational improvement. Short-term cost reductions can lead to customers' dissatisfaction, lower revenues, and decreased market share. In

Figure 22. Flattening the Hierarchy.

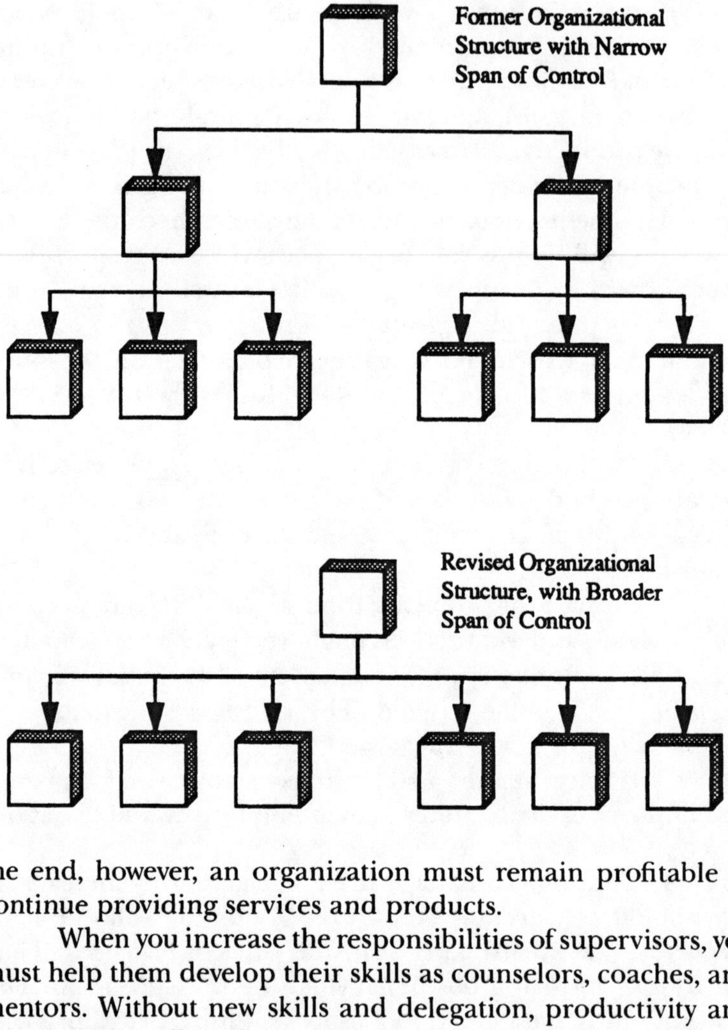

Former Organizational
Structure with Narrow
Span of Control

Revised Organizational
Structure, with Broader
Span of Control

the end, however, an organization must remain profitable to continue providing services and products.

When you increase the responsibilities of supervisors, you must help them develop their skills as counselors, coaches, and mentors. Without new skills and delegation, productivity and morale will suffer. Managers will also quickly burn out and become ineffective.

Action Step: **Develop approved methods of accomplishing each process.**

After making system improvements, define specific methods of performing each process and activity. This is time-consuming and may sound unnecessary; but without specified methods, how can you train people consistently to conduct their activities? Variation increases and quality decreases if employees do not all use the same methods.

Skilled employees should be used in designing methods. These people can contribute years of experience and perform activities in the most effective manner. Potential impacts of any process changes on other functions should be reviewed, particularly where other departments or programs are concerned. If approval of a method is required, it should be obtained. Use the approved methods to train current and new staff members.

Action Step: **Review and revise measurement criteria.**

Measurement criteria should be reviewed and revised under at least two conditions. First, criteria should be reviewed after any system improvement. Criteria may become irrelevant or even misleading after a system has been changed. New measurement criteria may now be relevant. Criteria should also be reviewed periodically to determine whether they are still useful. If they are not, discontinue them. Their only value is in assisting job performance or management.

Action Step: **Develop guidelines or standards for measures.**

This is an optional step. Now and only now is the time for considering guidelines or standards. Standards have no relevance if a function or output is no longer required, or if there are no approved methods for performing activities. This action is optional because there are two different philosophies about standards. In traditional management and industrial engineering, specific goals and standards are considered necessary for managers and employees to know what is expected of them. This approach has been used for many years. More recently, Deming (1986) has said that quotas or standards should not be used, and that numerical quotas should be eliminated. The most important point, however, is not whether goals or standards exist but how they are used. Standards or ratios are important for planning and scheduling. If the volume of work were to increase, how much more in staff time and supplies would be required? If other changes were made, what would the impacts be?

The primary objection of Deming and others to the use of standards is that they can be used as goals to evaluate individuals, especially without planning how to accomplish those goals. Whether or not standards are used, employees must understand how to do their jobs. If goals are used, then system or process changes for accomplishment *must* accompany them. It is most important to gain agreement on and develop an understanding of the process improvements; it is less important to have goals or standards. If standards or goals are used, however, they should be used for planning and scheduling rather than individual evaluation, be recognized as short-term guidelines until further process improvements are made, and be agreed to by the employees and managers involved.

Standards may provide useful milestones, but in themselves they do not improve processes. It is more cost-effective to concentrate efforts on improving processes. Industrial engineering methods (such as time study, time measurement, and work sampling) can be used to measure performance and determine standards.

Action Step: **Develop and implement performance monitoring and reporting.**

To evaluate common and special causes of variation and to determine the impacts of process changes, performance must be measured. A regular system of collecting and reporting measurements is useful in monitoring performance and identifying opportunities for improvement. Information about how well you are meeting customers' requirements and the organization's goals is always needed.

A monitoring system should collect and report actual values over time (and compare them with expected values, goals, or standards, if these are used). A reporting system should include all aspects of performance: work load, staffing, productivity, quality, utilization, and budget. It should provide for different levels of aggregation appropriate to the people reviewing the data. It should include data from several periods. Finally, it should provide for exception reporting, to identify items that need attention (such as points beyond control limits and runs of data).

Graphs illustrating information over time are relatively more useful to managers than tables of data because they are better at illustrating trends and patterns over time. Reporting of data for a single point in time should be avoided. Such information leads to inappropriate questions and decisions. (The use of quantitative information is discussed in more detail in Chapter Eleven.)

Action Step: **Ask basic questions about performance.**

When information becomes available, employees and managers should ask a series of questions to understand potential improvements:

1. What happened?
   - Did work loads increase or decrease?
   - Did productivity go up or down?
   - Did quality and service levels increase or decrease?
   - Is the process stable? (*Stability* is defined as an unchanged process generating the measurements. Instability is indicated by specific values far from the average of other values; downward or upward trends; and runs of points below average, above average, upward, or downward. Other patterns may also indicate that a process is not stable. The concept of stability is further explained in Deming, 1986.)
   - How did productivity compare to the standard?

2. Why did it happen? (Analysis of data by potential cause over time is necessary to answer these questions.)

- What were the reasons for the changes?
- What are the special causes of variation? (If the process is unstable, look for reasons causing the large deviations from the average or trends.)
- What are the common causes of variation? (If the process is stable, look for common characteristics of the process that explain variation from the desired performance.)

3. What are you going to do about it? (After forming theories or hypotheses to explain the observed performance, you will need to analyze the information to determine whether your theories or hypotheses are useful. An action plan for change, with measures to determine if improvements occur, should be developed.)

Action Step: **Manage resources to match work load and demand.**

One of the most effective methods of improving cost-effectiveness is to manage resources to match the work load or demand, which is accomplished through several approaches.

The first approach is to manage the demand or work load. Patients' visits to a nurse practitioner are scheduled to ensure that the nurse remains busy. Scheduling can also help reduce the waiting time of patients or other customers. Ask questions: Can the work load be eliminated? Is it unnecessary? Can the work load be transferred elsewhere, for improved overall productivity or lower costs? (Any such transfer, of course, must be reasonable and mutually agreeable to the parties involved.) Can the arrival or service time be scheduled? If so, what are customers' requirements and constraints? Can the work load be prioritized by the time required? (For example, a secretary receives a number of requests for work — some required today, some required later. If time requirements are specified, work can be prioritized by the time required.)

Whether you can schedule the work load or not, it is useful to predict when it will occur. Past data can be used to predict the approximate magnitude and timing of future demand. Analysis of patients' arrivals at an emergency room can be used to estimate the future number of arrivals by severity level, hour of the day, and day of the week. Since emergencies are unscheduled, such predictions are seldom completely correct, but they can be used to schedule staff and other resources to improve cost-effectiveness.

Better matching of staff, supplies, and other resources to the work load will improve cost-effectiveness. Scheduling is best, and prediction is second best, but other methods should also be used when they are appropriate—for example, transferring staff among different job functions to meet the high-priority demand, requesting overtime, calling staff in to meet high-unplanned-demand periods, scheduling vacations and time off during periods of low demand, and asking staff to go home if there is inadequate demand. In the latter case, staff may be given partial pay if they go home. Overall, costs would still be reduced. Variable budgeting is another useful method of focusing attention on matching staff and other resources to the work load, whether up or down.

Chapter Eleven

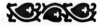

Managing with Quantitative and Qualitative Information

This chapter describes how to improve cost-effectiveness through the use of quantitative and qualitative management information. With the increased complexity of clinical care, financing and regulatory requirements, and the structure of healthcare organizations themselves, effective use of information has become much more important.

Hospitals spend substantial amounts of time and money on information processing, but comparatively less than other information-intensive organizations. According to Zinn and DiGiulio (1988, p. 32), "Recent surveys indicate that hospitals spend approximately 3 percent of their operating budget for data processing costs—almost $4.5 billion each year. Other studies show that fully one-third of all tasks within the health-care setting are related to managing information—over $25 billion annually." Other information-intensive organizations, such as banks, spend approximately double this percentage of their budgets on formal information-processing functions. Greater increases are predicted to be spent on information management in the future.

Hospitals, more than other types of healthcare providers, tend to spend a larger percentage of their budgets on information management, but recent surveys also show increases in other provider organizations.

Focus of Quantitative Information

Both the focus and the scope of quantitative information have changed dramatically in the last few years. Twenty years ago, most organizations involved with healthcare were internally focused. This was equally true of hospitals, nursing homes, physicians, insurance companies, federal and state agencies, and businesses paying for healthcare insurance. Healthcare providers primarily waited until a patient arrived, and then they maintained information on that episode of care and filed the information later. Likewise, third-party payers collected little summary information for management decisions. Except in medical research, little use was made of the information after the patient was discharged. Today the environment is competitive and financially risky for everyone, and most organizations maintain much more information, as a way of understanding their own operations, their competitors, and their environments.

Increased competition in the healthcare industry affects all organizations and has led to increased information requirements. For example, hospitals are competing on price and quality, not just in their local markets but nationally. The state of California began a process of having hospitals bid to provide care to MediCal (California Medicaid) patients. A number of medical centers are now offering fixed discount prices for selected specialty care (such as coronary bypass surgery). A major academic health center has now become a national center for coronary bypass surgery. Its prices, even with air fare and patients' and families' accommodations, are still lower than those of many local medical centers. Large business organizations are also requesting competitive bids from insurance companies and offer their employees several different choices at different out-of-pocket costs, and hospitals and nursing homes with low occupancies are offering discounts in their transitional inpatient units, which cost much less than continued acute care. As a consequence, the focus, scope, and use of information have increased dramatically. Here are some examples of information changes:

1. *External customer information*: To promote better understanding of customers' needs, detailed demographic, healthcare-use, and opinion information is collected and ana-

lyzed by healthcare providers, HMOs, insurance companies, and federal and state agencies.

2. *Information on competitors*: Detailed information on facilities, services, interprovider relationships, customers, customers' perceptions, quality measures, costs, and plans is collected and analyzed as a way of understanding the status and plans of competitors. Information on competitors fosters better decisions and creates a competitive advantage.

3. *Internal customers' requirements*: These customers and their requirements are being defined, to improve the quality of services provided within the organization and, ultimately, to improve services to external customers.

4. *Internal service and cost information*: Detailed information is being collected on specific services as well as costs. Information-collection systems have different names and uses and can evaluate services and costs at many different levels of detail.

5. *Information on external vendors and costs*: Information on current and competing vendors' products and services, prices, features, and quality is important in decisions about products and vendors.

More detailed information is being collected and used by all organizations. This is being made possible by large computers and data-base software.

> *Action Step*: **Verify that your information system can address in detail at least the following: your customers, your competitors, your suppliers, competitors of your suppliers, and alternative sources. For high-volume or high-cost items, the competition will be regional, national, or even international.**

Performance Measurement

This section provides an approach to measuring performance. The information is intended for leaders and managers;

we avoid the specific details of how systems for performance measurement work.

Components of Performance Measurement

Performance measurement involves quantitative evaluation of all aspects of the healthcare system. It is not limited to productivity. Performance measurement should include at least the following aspects of your business.

Mission and Goals. Performance measurement should address the mission, values, and goals of the organization or department. If measurement does not address the goals, one of two things will happen: progress toward meeting goals will not be addressed or, worse, you will measure and focus attention on topics contrary to the goals.

Work Load or Outputs. Since work load drives your resource requirements, it is necessary to measure and monitor your work loads.

Resource or Process Capabilities. The types of resources and processes you use will affect outcomes and therefore should be measured. Examples of these are staff credentials and the kinds of information you use from medical records.

Resources Used or Inputs. For healthcare organizations, the most important resource is people. Time used by category of staff is an important measure, but other limited and costly resources are also used, such as facilities, equipment, medications, supplies, and dollars.

Productivity. This is the ratio of resource inputs to workload outputs. Generally, these are calculated individually (for example, the number of nursing hours per inpatient day).

Quality- or Service-Level Measures. These gauge how well a service meets the customers' requirements. High productivity has little value if you provide poor service.

Utilization. This is a measure of the percentage of a resource used versus the amount available. For example, the percentage of inpatient occupancy is the number of beds used for patients, divided by the total number of beds available for use.

Financial Performance. Costs, revenues, and net income are very important to a healthcare organization. Without profits, there is no money to change or develop new services, products, or information. The budget converts all of the services provided and resources used into dollars and then compares actual dollar revenues and expenditures with the expected revenues and expenditures.

Each type of measurement provides different quantitative information to healthcare managers. If measures for one or more of the components are missing, those areas will be inadequately addressed. Clinical and nonclinical measures should both be included.

> ***Action Step***: **Review your system of performance measurement to determine whether measures exist for all key components. If not, add them.**

Context of Performance Measurement

Performance is generally measured in one or more contexts within an organization or entity. Most of the components of performance measurement can apply to each of the places to measure performance: outputs, intermediate services and products, processes, and inputs.

Outputs. These are the services and products we provide to our patients and other customers and are the reason for our existence. Sample outputs are outpatient physician visits, surgical procedures, pharmacy prescriptions, inpatient diagnosis-related groups (DRGs), inpatient days of care, mortality and morbidity rates resulting from care, and days of posthospitalization recovery before returning to work.

Intermediate Services and Products. These are services or products produced to support the basic outputs. Examples include laundry, meals, medical records, maintenance, and housekeeping.

Process. Performance is often evaluated by comparing the actual process of providing services and products with a desired or expected process. An example is verification that care provided to a patient is documented in the medical record, and that the record is signed by the appropriate care providers.

Inputs. These are measurements of people, other resources, or customers at the time they enter a healthcare system or the particular encounter. Such measurements ensure that the different inputs meet the requirements considered necessary for a successful outcome. Examples include credentialing of physicians and nurses, inspection of incoming supplies, and preadmission testing of patients.

All of the types of measurements are useful, but the output measurements are particularly important because they directly measure the outcomes of our efforts for our customers.

Transaction Data Versus Management Information

Many current computer systems in healthcare organizations are focused on data to complete a transaction and provide little information useful for management to measure or improve the process. A pharmacy transaction can serve as an example. A physician writes an order for medication. That information is entered into a pharmacy computer system, which produces a label, and the medication is prepared by the pharmacist. When the medication is administered or issued, that fact is entered into the computer, and the computer may create a patient charge. The medication may even be subtracted from inventory, and new medications may be ordered when the stock is diminished. The system supports the medication transaction, but few such systems provide any cumulative management information. For example, what is the level of medication use by patients in specific DRGs? What are the type, amount, and value of the medication that has been administered to a patient or type of patient over time? This type of management information is becoming critically important as resource constraints become more severe. Physicians and other healthcare professionals need this information for evaluating potential changes in clinical practices. Managers need this type of information for evaluating process improvements.

Criteria and Standards

Whether standards are used or not, it is necessary to measure performance. Definitions vary by user, and so it is necessary to state your definitions. As you would expect, different organizations use terms differently, but the concepts are similar. Although often ignored, definitions also vary substantially within a single organization. The following terms are used in this book.

Criterion. This is a variable that is measured and reported (worked hours per patient day on a nursing unit, waiting time in an outpatient service, customers' opinion about courtesy of service). Some use the term *parameter* instead of criterion.

Standard. This is the value of the criterion. In a nursing unit, the standard might be 5.5 worked hours per patient day. The term *standard* is used loosely in the healthcare industry, and several different words are considered to be synonymous:

1. *Norm:* This is a less precise term, used to refer to a median, average, or other guideline, imprecisely defined or from imprecise sources.
2. *Guideline:* This is an agreed-upon expectation of perfor-

mance with which actual performance is compared. It is similar to a standard but has a less scientific connotation.

3. *Mean or average*: This is the numerical mean, or average, of a criterion from a specified sample or group.

4. *Median*: This is the midpoint of a criterion from a specified sample or group. *MONITREND*, a publication of the American Hospital Association, publishes median values of many criteria for different groups of hospitals.

5. *Standard*: This is a criterion or benchmark with which actual performance is compared. A standard may apply to staff time, quality, or any other variable.

6. *Time Standard*: This is the time determined to be necessary for a qualified person, working at a pace ordinarily used under capable supervision and experiencing normal fatigue and delays, to do a defined amount of work of specified quality while following the prescribed method.

You need not know these definitions by heart, but be aware of the following cautions. All of these are called *standards* in different settings. A true time standard includes several critically important components: prescribed method, qualified person, ordinary pace, capable supervision, and normal fatigue and delays. You first must understand what you are trying to accomplish: planning, scheduling, or evaluation. Then you must ask the definition and the source of the standards before you can use them appropriately. Each of the preceding definitions is useful for certain purposes. Some people tend to overstate the validity and usefulness of standards. The different engineering methods used to establish standards are addressed in many reference documents (for example, Maynard, 1971).

Selected sources of comparative standards, medians, and guidelines are listed here. These are often appropriate for identifying potential opportunities for improvement, but they are occasionally used inappropriately, as in setting goals without any method for achieving them:

- *MONITREND* reports medians of many criteria for hospitals of different sizes, case-mix intensities, and teaching affiliation.

- Resource Monitoring System (RMS) gives measured standards for activities of several different hospital departments.
- Methods Time Measurement (MTM) can be used to develop predetermined elemental times that can be summed to develop activity standards.
- Professional Activity Study (PAS), from the Commission on Professional and Hospital Activities, gives comparative statistics related to medical care that are useful for quality evaluation and utilization review.
- The Joint Commission on Accreditation of Healthcare Organizations gives standards related to practice and processes in hospitals, nursing homes, and other organizations.
- Proprietary standards are available through most consulting companies working in the healthcare industry.

Whatever method is chosen, those using it must understand its value and weaknesses. Methods should be used as tools, not as definitive measures or answers. Remember, the large majority of performance improvements occur through process improvements, and standards by themselves do not accomplish process improvements.

> *Action Step*: **Decide whether and how standards will be used in your organization, and communicate that decision. If standards will be used for evaluation, extreme caution should be taken to ensure that there are agreed-upon methods to achieve the goals and that the goals are acceptable to the employees.**

Development of a Quantitative Information System

Developing a good quantitative information system is an iterative process. The process is complicated by changing information, as well as by computer systems and the shortage of people knowledgeable about their availability and use. If you were to calculate and distribute detailed costs for every clinical procedure provided by your organization, few if any managers would have any idea what to do with the information. Therefore, the data would not be used. By contrast, if you asked managers to identify useful information, they would be limited by their current roles and knowledge and might not identify all the relevant useful information.

General Requirements

Regardless of how an information system is developed, the following requirements or general guidelines are key to any quantitative information system.

Information Use. The use of information is the primary reason for developing a quantitative information system. The quality of information that is not used deteriorates quickly because no one has an interest in its validity.

Computerization. Given the magnitude of information required, as well as the need to integrate information from different sources, computerization of the data is most cost-effective. This is particularly true for information used more than once. Manually collected, stored, and analyzed data are most useful for circumstances in which the data will not be required again.

Data-Base Structure. Given current technology, a large data-base structure is the most effective way to handle large amounts of information. A data base allows different data to be easily related, combined, and reported.

Compatibility and Communication. Your different computer hardware, software, and data files should be compatible and capable of communicating with one another. It is impractical and unnecessary to plan one "supercomputer" system to receive, process, and produce all the information required. The important characteristic is that files on one computer system should be able to be accessed and used by other computer systems.

Data-Element Administration. Even if data can be moved from one computer to another, the information has little use unless its elements are compatible and have the same operational definitions. A data-element description includes the definition (common, professional, specific, local), field size, type of field (alphabetical, numerical, alphanumerical, compacted), range or acceptable set of values, calculation method (if applicable), cross reference(s) to other data elements, use or application, constraints, abbreviation, person responsible for data element, and date approved. Someone should be responsible for the administration of data elements, to ensure common definitions and uses.

Cost Benefits of Information. Collecting, storing, and reporting information costs money. The benefits of information must be compared with its costs. One difficulty in evaluating the cost benefits of information is the unknown future implications of that information. This is not an argument for collecting data with no known use; rather, it is a recognition that information used for one purpose today may be important for another purpose in the future.

Access and Security. All large computer systems have mechanisms to address access and security. To a degree, there is a trade-off between allowing access and providing for security and privacy of information.

Flexibility. Our information requirements continue to expand and change. Therefore, the flexibility to change in the future is a key system requirement. That is also a key reason for using a large data base.

Intelligence or Internal Checking. The capability for both syntax and logical checking of input data and other types of intelligence should be planned into all mainframe computer programs.

Backup or Contingency System. With our increasing dependence on computerized information systems comes increased risk of a major system failure. Backup and contingency plans should provide for large-scale power shortages, catastrophic computer failure, and so on. The healthcare system must continue to function. Healthcare services are particularly critical if a power shortage is caused by a natural disaster involving widespread injury.

Considerations for Development of an Information System

Developing an effective quantitative information system is an iterative undertaking, but what process should be used? While there is no one best approach, the following considerations are important.

Current System Requirements. The current information system, whatever its advantages and problems, is a starting place. Even if new computer hardware and software are acquired, the data in the new system must be related to your current system.

Payers' Requirements. Medicare, Medicaid, Blue Cross, health maintenance organizations, and other payers are imposing more and more information requirements. Meeting these requirements is essential to receiving reimbursements, whether by computerized or manual methods. To the extent possible, payers' requirements should be integrated into the regular computerized information system.

Local, Regional, and National Cooperative Data Bases. Hospital associations, nursing home associations, other professional associations, and state and federal agencies request information for evaluation and reporting. These are sources of comparative information.

Clinical Programs and Product Lines. Data s'iould be sufficient and suitable for summary by clinical programs and product lines. Multidisciplinary and multi-institutional clinical programs and product lines are becoming common and will continue to increase as healthcare providers focus on customers' requirements. Physicians' information requirements will also be integrated with the requirements of hospitals, nursing homes, and home-care agencies as systems of continuing care expand.

Customer-Based Data. Through both quality-improvement efforts and market competition, healthcare providers and related organizations require much better customer-based information for marketing, service development, and evaluation.

Clinical Requirements. Physicians, nurses, and other care providers are integrating computerized information into patient care, management, evaluation, research, and education activities. Medical centers, for example, are offering on-line computer connections to community physicians' offices, to provide information, schedule patients, and provide education.

Management Requirements. Cost-effectiveness, as described in Chapter Ten, is of critical importance to healthcare providers, payers, industry and business corporations, state and federal agencies, and other organizations. Detailed information is required for appropriate management decisions.

Any quantitative information system is a compromise of technical, operational, and economic factors. All of the considerations just discussed affect decisions on which type of information system to develop.

> *Action Step*: **Verify that you are meeting the general requirements of an information system and that your system provides information both to complete service transactions and to manage the processes involved.**

Management Decisions with Quantitative Information

Few management decisions today can be made safely without quantitative information. Industrial and business corporations and payers are doing everything possible to reduce their healthcare costs. We have argued that all organizations involved with healthcare today are at increased risk. Because financial and other resources are limited, healthcare organizations cannot do everything they would like to do. Therefore, information is essential, to quantify current and potential situations, to set priorities for alternatives, and to make informed decisions. Some approaches and examples are described here, to illustrate how leaders and managers can utilize quantitative information effectively in decision making.

Business-Plan Approach. A complete business plan is necessary for fully informed decisions. Most proposals submitted for decisions are incomplete. When physicians, managers, and others propose new services, products, facilities, or equipment, a complete business plan should be required. The plan does not have to be lengthy, but it should address the following types of topics:

I. Purpose/Objectives
II. Summary
III. Service and/or Product Description
IV. Work Load
    A. Work-Load Measures
    B. Projected Volume(s)
    C. Basis and/or Source of Work-Load Projections
        1. Source Documents
        2. Marketing Analysis
        3. Appropriateness of Use
    D. Related Work Loads and Changes
        1. Changes in Functions, Operation, and/or Responsibilities
        2. Ancillary Departmental Work-Load Changes
        3. Supporting Departmental Work-Load Changes
        4. Return Business (for example, inpatient admission leads to follow-up outpatient care)
V. Revenue

    A.   Components of Revenue (for example, pricing)
    B.   Projected Incremental Revenues
    C.   Reimbursement Impact
       1.   Payer Mix for Services and Products Being Affected
       2.   Payer Contract Limitations
       3.   Net Payments Received

VI.   Costs
    A.   Incremental Changes in Operating Costs (annual, monthly)
       1.   Current Staffing and Productivity
       2.   Ability of Current Staff to Absorb Changes in Work Load (for example, impact on productivity, service, quality)
       3.   Changes in Number and Skill Mix of Staff
       4.   Changes in Organization and Management
       5.   Nonlabor Resource Changes (facilities, equipment, supplies)
       6.   Components of Costs (labor, commodities, equipment, facilities) and Estimated Costs
    B.   Start-Up/Implementation Costs
       1.   Components of Costs
          a.   Labor (including training)
          b.   Commodities (supplies and nonlabor costs)
             (1)   Capital Equipment
             (2)   Facility Changes
       2.   Estimated Costs
       3.   Sources of Funds

VII.   Marginal Changes/Contribution
    A.   Financial Contribution
       1.   Annual Contribution or Margin
       2.   Return on Investment
    B.   Quality/Service-Level Changes
    C.   Educational Impacts
    D.   Research Impacts
    E.   Other Changes (for example, market position)

VIII. Implementation Plan

      A.   Actions Required (give list of major actions)
      B.   Person/People Responsible
      C.   Schedule
         1.   Milestone Dates
         2.   Possibly Time or Gantt Chart
IX.   Performance Monitoring
      A.   Monitoring Criteria
         1.   Goals
         2.   Work Load/Outputs
         3.   Resources/Inputs
         4.   Productivity
         5.   Quality/Service Level
         6.   Utilization Review
         7.   Budget
      B.   System to Monitor Performance
X.   Deactivation Plan If Projections Do Not Occur
      A.   Review Date for Implementation
      B.   Review Criteria

Not all of this information is relevant to every decision. Long-term commitments to programs, facilities, contracts, and so on can have major consequences for your organization's financial viability. Too often, commitments are made without serious evaluation of the costs and benefits of a proposal.

> *Action Step*: **Use a business-plan approach in considering data for all major decisions. A plan need not be extremely detailed for some decisions.**

Performance Monitoring. Regular monitoring of performance is necessary in identifying and acting on changes in a timely manner and keeping people informed. Performance monitoring requires a set of measurements, a reporting system, management action, and possibly a set of performance expectations, or standards. Using the components of and context for performance monitoring just described, each function or department should have multiple criteria for measuring different aspects of performance. Information should be shared with all involved managers and employees. Employees should be provided with reports on utilization and other performance (Solovy, 1988b). Monitoring must also extend beyond your organization. Customers' perceptions and requirements, competitors' capabilities and performance, and environmental changes must be monitored to support management decisions.

The use of performance expectations, or standards, is subject to some debate, although virtually everyone advocates measuring performance. Most professionals advocate the use of some level of expectation, if not specific standards, for each reporting period (day, week, month). Numerical quotas tend to lead to either low quality (induced by the staff's meeting unreasonable quotas) or lower than optimal productivity (because staff members quit when they reach the quota). We advocate regular measurement, with short-term, changing goals or expectations for performance instead of the more rigidly interpreted standards. Goals for quality should take priority over volume or productivity goals.

A reporting system is then developed, to report actual performance measurements and goals, if used. The following characteristics are useful in a reporting system:

1. *Varying levels of detail*: The level of detail required to evaluate and improve performance varies with the level of management. Hence, a reporting system should provide summary reports for senior managers, with detailed reports for section or department managers.
2. *Format*: To provide a balanced picture of performance, the report should include a trend (or run) chart of multiple performance measurements. Graphs with control limits are very useful in detecting the need for action.
3. *Frequency*: As with level of detail, the frequency of reports will depend on the action required. To manage daily activities in a production area (such as dietetics), measurement should be made several times per day. For overall budget management, monthly reports are appropriate.
4. *Method of computation*: It is best if performance monitoring is tied to the computerized financial system, so that data are

regularly collected and directly related to financial reports. Various systems are available on microcomputers, minicomputers, and mainframe computers. Even if data are manually collected and summarized, however, regular performance monitoring is important.

Variable Budgeting. An extension of performance monitoring is to develop variable budgets based on work loads. The budget for any given month is then based on the volume of each variable work load, multiplied by the staff time and resources required to perform that work load. These figures are then converted to a dollar budget. Finally, any fixed staff, resource, and budget figures are added, to determine the total expected budget for the month. Thus, the budget will automatically go up and down with the work load. This approach, also called *flexible budgeting*, is consistent with the concept of maintaining constant productivity for staff and other resources.

Management with Qualitative Information

Quantitative information should be complemented by qualitative information. Quantitative information is certainly useful in managing current operations and even in providing external information about patients and other customers, competitors, vendors, and so on. Since most quantitative information is based on past experience, it is useful whenever past experience can be used to make current decisions or predict the future. Quantitative information is seldom of any real use, however, when major new markets or paradigm shifts in society must be predicted. The faster and more dramatic a change, the less useful historical quantitative information is. The following examples illustrate this point:

1. When the lithotripter was introduced for crushing kidney stones without surgery, the number of surgical procedures for kidney stones dropped sharply.
2. When the drug cimetidine, sold under the brand name of

Tagamet, was introduced for controlling ulcers, the number of surgical procedures for ulcers dropped sharply.

3. The use of lasers for ophthalmological procedures has radically changed care and shifted procedures to ambulatory clinics, decreasing the use of inpatient beds.

4. When Medicare began reimbursing for inpatient care on the basis of DRGs, this practice radically changed financial incentives, clinical practices, and the use of healthcare services in a way that could not have been predicted by historical data.

5. Closure of a large industrial plant in a community will cause declines in the local population, economy, and demand for healthcare services.

6. Even the most sophisticated computerized models were unable to predict the crash of the stock market in October 1987.

Leaders must make a continual effort to seek out quantitative information that signals major changes in social expectations, clinical practice, and the economy. These changes represent the greatest potential if they are predicted and acted on and the greatest risk if they are not predicted or acted on.

Action Step: **Actively pursue qualitative and quantitative information that signals major changes in social expectations, clinical practice, and the economy. This information will not be available from your organization's current quantitative data.**

Healthcare leaders should look at the following types of qualitative information, to supplement the available quantitative information:

- Social expectations and trends
- Pending legislation (federal, state, or local)
- Changing clinical practices

- Clinical research, which can affect the need for healthcare services or healthcare delivery methods
- Potential new services that may affect healthcare
- Plans of industrial corporations in the area
- Plans of healthcare organizations in the area
- New sports or social activities

Social research groups and others quantify some of these opinions and trends and can provide information to supplement what is normally used in healthcare organizations.

Training and Personnel Development

It should be clear that everyone in your organization will have to be trained to work more effectively with quantitative information. Ideally, training should be tailored to the current and planned activities of each person. With the resources currently available to most organizations, however, such individualized instruction is unrealistic. Employees, medical staff, and others accessing the information should therefore be trained in groups that require similar information. In the future, use of computerized training modules will allow each employee to receive training tailored to his or her needs and interests.

Chapter Twelve

Rethinking Strategies for Leadership Effectiveness

Frames of reference for definitions and requirements of leadership are constantly changing. The perceived importance of leadership is also evolving. Much more than in the past, leadership is a key determinant of whether an organization prospers or fails. In this chapter, we present different definitions of leadership and propose a fresh approach. To achieve major transformation, leaders who promote and celebrate change are required at all levels in an organization, as opposed to managers who focus on maintaining the status quo. A brief historical description of healthcare management may be helpful in illustrating why we believe that a new approach is necessary.

The early role for a healthcare administrator was to keep the medical staff happy and to provide an environment and staffing to support the care prescribed by physicians. Most staff and management energy was devoted to completing the transaction of physicians' orders. Since the goal was to maintain the status quo, little information was collected or used for learning better methods or improving processes, and there was no incentive to be cost-efficient.

The role of management was considered for a long time to include five components. Mackenzie (1969, pp. 80–87) describes them as planning ("predetermine a course of action"); organizing ("arrange and relate work for effective accomplishment of objectives"); coordinating ("choose competent people for positions in [the] organization," and integrate and schedule all resources to accomplish results); directing ("bring about purposeful action toward desired objectives"); and controlling ("ensure progress toward objectives according to [the] plan").

While these skills are important, we believe that there has been inappropriate emphasis on the directing and controlling aspects of management. The approach to implementation has been authoritative and has ignored the human elements of the organization — namely, the fact that the person doing the work is in the best position to recommend ways for the process to be improved. Managers in the past were correct in treating physicians as customers, but they ignored the importance of other internal and external customers.

Leaders Versus Managers

Leader, manager, administrator, and other terms are used in many different contexts and have many different definitions. The point of this discussion is to distinguish the skills and behaviors of typical leaders from those of traditional managers of administrators. There is no single set of requirements for a leader, nor is there anyone who exhibits all the characteristics.

There are several distinctions between typical leaders and managers. Managers have been described as people who maintain the operations of an organization, relate to others according to the organizational structure, and seek acceptable compromises among conflicting priorities. The main point is that managers frequently identify with the current organization and seek to maintain the status quo. Their relationships with others are characterized as impersonal and detached. Managers tend to exhibit impersonal attitudes and view specific goals as means of getting the job done. In contrast, leaders are dissatisfied with the status quo; they imagine new areas to explore and create new approaches. Leaders relate to people in more intuitive and empathetic ways and can excite people with their visions of the future. They are willing to take risks where opportunities and rewards are high. Leaders are active. They shape ideas, rather than responding to them. They adopt a personal and active attitude toward goals, and they change the way people think about what is desirable, possible, and necessary. Where managers seek to limit choices, leaders develop fresh approaches to long-standing problems, and they open issues for new options (Zaleznek, 1977).

Bennis and Nanus (1985, p. 21) have articulated another useful perspective in differentiating between leading and managing: "To manage means to bring about, to accomplish, to have charge of or responsibility for, to conduct. . . . Leading is influencing, guiding in direction, course, action, opinion. . . . Managers are people who do things right and leaders are people who do the right thing."

Burns (1978, p. 4) identifies two basic types of leadership, the *transactional* and the *transforming*: "The relations of most leaders and followers are transactional; leaders approach followers with an eye to exchanging one thing for another; jobs for votes, or subsidies for campaign contributions. Transforming leadership, while more complex, is more potent. The transforming leader recognizes and exploits an existing need or demand of a potential follower. But, beyond that, the transforming leader looks for potential motives in followers, seeks to satisfy higher needs, and engages the full person of the follower. The result of the transforming leadership is a relationship of mutual stimulation and elevation that converts followers into leaders and may convert leaders into moral agents." With the lack of faith in healthcare administration now being expressed by the American public, this transforming leadership is the type our industry needs now.

Table 5 contrasts characteristics of successful leaders with characteristics of nondynamic managers. The contrast is of personal characteristics, and the way the person operates, rather than a reflection of a person's job title.

When resources are plentiful, when reimbursement is adequate, and when competition is minimal, profitability is virtually ensured. Under these circumstances, organizations have little need for leadership. Particularly from 1965 through 1985, the "golden era" of healthcare, almost all organizations in the industry did well. There was little need for leadership of the type we are describing. Because of stability in the industry, most healthcare managers focused on transactions that maintained current business; little or no attention was given to basic

Table 5. Characteristics of Leaders Versus Managers.

Characteristics of Successful Leaders for the Future, Including Transformational Leaders	*Characteristics of Nondynamic Managers, Including Transactional Leaders*
Focuses externally; is market- or community-oriented	Focuses internally
Builds large external networks	Builds minimal external networks
Visits customers and suppliers	Focuses on internal work
Measures progress against competitors	Measures progress against last year
Notices small market changes	Notices only large market changes
Acts as a change agent	Maintains the status quo
Creates and communicates a vision and values	Conveys no vision for the future
Is committed to learning change	Keeps options open
Articulates values to employees	Assumes that employees know the values
Understands and motivates people	Directs people
Shares information with employees	Guards information
Delegates responsibility and authority	Centralizes authority
Seeks new ideas and changes	Avoids changes
Mobilizes the organization toward a vision	
Views education and training as investments in human capital	Views education and training as expenses

changes. For example, an insurance company's account manager could focus all his or her attention on processing paper bills rather than on investigating new ways of communicating.

Other than the addition of high technology, there have been few changes in the way care is delivered to patients. Systems of care provision are very traditional. This situation brings to mind the statement that managers spend time tinkering with systems that are rotten to the core. Our systems need major revamping. We must challenge both systems and processes, to see what can be simplified or deleted, and we must examine the processes that support patients' care. An example of how to change a process to improve the delivery of care is being provided in Japan, at Tokai University Hospital. Quality experts are recording the conversations of nurses with patients during such procedures as admitting in order to analyze, with quantitative data based on linguistic theory, the therapeutic value of the nurses' words. The nurses then get feedback on how to improve the therapeutic quality of interactions (Morooka, 1989). We do many things in healthcare because we have always done them that way. By thinking creatively about the work that needs to be accomplished and designing processes anew from the bottom up, there is much that we can do to improve our quality, productivity, and cost-efficiency.

Skills and Knowledge Necessary for Transformation

The type of leader necessary in these times is one who can build on the apparent strengths of the organization and teach people how to function more efficiently and effectively. This new-age leader demonstrates many of the old skills but also has a repertoire of new ones.

Being a Visionary. A new-age leader must be a visionary. Tapping into the vast knowledge of the front-line employee requires a leader who can create a new vision for the organization that will empower, inspire, and enable people to improve the workplace. This must occur "in the midst of a perpetual competitive hurricane to encourage people to take day-to-day risks involved in testing and adopting and extending the vision" (Peters, 1987, p. 485).

Visioning is much more than conjuring up a visual image. It is a skill that you can develop with practice. Think about any situation, and imagine it in full detail. Describe what you see, feel, and hear. You should envision a technicolor picture of future potential.

It may be helpful to begin by using this skill to flesh out a personal issue before you move to visioning in a business situation. Suppose that you wish to lose ten pounds. Visioning can help you achieve the goal. To begin, select a free time of day and a place where you will not be interrupted. Sit in a comfortable chair and take some deep breaths to relax. Concentrate on your breathing for a few seconds. Then think about your goal. What could you look like in two months? What would the benefits of weight loss be? Would there be any disadvantages? Whom can you count on to support you? Who will set up barriers? How can you reduce or deal with those barriers?

When you move to develop a vision related to business, you use the same approach and ask the same types of questions. Think about the ideal future for your organization or department. What steps are necessary for you to accomplish the vision? What barriers would keep you from achieving your goals? What actions would reduce those barriers? "Listening, reading, smelling, feeling, and tasting the business improves our vision" (Kouzes and Posner, 1987, p. 95). Think about your vision often. Focus on it clearly, affirm it, and continue to press for implementation. Leaders must look to the future and express a clear, long-term strategy for the journey. Making a vision a reality by attracting people to it is also the role of the leader.

Action Step: **Practice visioning skills for planning purposes. Consider both personal and professional goals as opportunities.**

Being Socially Responsible. Corporate social responsibility is important to meaningful leadership (Bisesi, 1983). Both as an individual and as a corporate leader, one should demonstrate social responsibility. In the past, it has been easier and cheaper for organizations to pollute the environment, abuse workers, ignore customers' requirements, and take other socially irresponsible actions. This is short-term thinking.

The conflict between declining resources and continuing social responsibility causes a real dilemma for healthcare leaders. You need to promote an attitude of social responsibility with respect to both the cost-effectiveness of services and products and the provision of services to those who cannot afford them. The trade-off of costs versus services must also be communicated. Ethical leadership will improve your relationship with the community you serve.

Action Step: **Discuss social responsibility of healthcare organizations at your management**

meetings. Give managers a chance to discuss major ethical issues.

Managing Uncertainty. A leader recognizes that nothing is certain and that all processes and outcomes are variable. According to Peters (1987, p. 474), "Today's successful business leaders will be those who are most flexible of mind. An ability to embrace new ideas, routinely challenge old ones, and live with paradox will be the effective leader's premier trait. Further, the challenge is for a lifetime. New truths will not emerge easily. Leaders will have to guide the ship while simultaneously putting everything up for grabs, which is itself a fundamental paradox."

Teach your staff to reduce variability. The important points are that the output of every process has variability and that a management decision should be based on an understanding of measurements over time, not on a single measurement.

Action Step: **Demand that managers and staff present graphs of data over several periods, not data for a single period.**

A security manager may request additional staff because of last month's large work load. Instead of making any decision on that single month's data, ask the security manager to bring you the work-load data for the last twelve to eighteen months. You can then see trends, single high or low points, and variations. If all the managers in your organization were to review graphs of data, instead of making decisions on the basis of single points, they would greatly improve their skills in managing uncertainty and variability. The other method of helping people to manage variability is to put less emphasis on measurements from a single time period.

Being a Change Agent. Leaders identify themselves as — and act as — change agents (Peters, 1987; Tichy and Devanna, 1986a). They should have a bias for action and an orientation toward constant improvement. They should spend much of their time eliminating barriers to change and improvement.

"The dominant culture in most big companies demands punishment for a mistake, no matter how useful, small, invisible" (Peters and Waterman, 1982, p. 48). Such an attitude tends to drive out change agents. To set the tone for improvement in your organization, make sure that you create the kind of atmosphere where your managers feel free to take risks and suggest change. Start meetings with an opportunity for people to discuss what they have changed since the last time you met. Continually ask yourself and your employees how every product and process can be improved or upgraded.

> *Action Step*: **Wander around the organization and ask employees what changes they have made in their units.**

Being People-Oriented. The leader must believe in people and should spend time acting as a coach and mentor, rather than as an evaluator and disciplinarian (Peters, 1987; Deming, 1986). The leader believes that people are the key to success and attracts followers by building trust and excitement. Help your organization be more people-oriented by modeling the behaviors you wish to see in the environment. Foster collaboration and teamwork. Emphasize the importance of long-term commitment; there are tremendous costs associated with turnover. You should emphasize your commitment to your employees.

> *Action Step*: **Lead by example. Encourage behaviors showing that people are your most important asset. Personally serve as a coach and mentor, and encourage those who work for you to do the same.**

> *Action Step*: **Encourage positive statements about your people in general, and discourage statements implying that people are easily replaceable or unimportant.**

Sharing Information. Some managers fear that sharing information will reduce their importance and power. Some new market plans certainly need to be closely guarded until the new service, facility, or product is introduced, but basic information on performance should be shared with all managers and staff members who are involved. For example, information on the work load, productivity, quality, utilization, and budget of the dietetics department should be shared with managers and employees in dietetics. In particular, employees should see performance measurements directly related to the areas in which they work. This attitude can be initiated through widespread sharing of information about work loads, customer surveys, quality measures, changes at competitors' institutions, overall financial status, and confirmed plans for the future.

> *Action Step*: **Ask managers what specific information is being shared with employees, look for performance data posted in departments throughout the organization, and ask specific employees what information is needed.**

Being Driven by Customers' Values. The leader clearly identifies current and potential customers and is driven to meet and exceed their expectations. Peters (1987) calls this characteristic *customer responsiveness*; Tichy and Devanna (1986a) refer to it as *value-driven management.* Leaders focus externally, rather than focusing all their attention on internal issues and problems.

To integrate the focus on customers into your management, use the vocabulary of customers and customers' requirements. Discussions related to all external and internal relationships should be considered customer-supplier relationships.

It may be unrealistic to visit every patient. Nevertheless, visit as many as possible during rounds, and ask about services. Ask what is working well and not so well, from the customer's perspective. Also visit internal customer departments and external business customers. To have a customer focus, you must stay in personal contact.

> *Action Step*: **Visit customers yourself, and request that other managers and key employees visit their**

customers and discuss their requirements. Ask about your services and products, and listen to the customers' comments and concerns. Remember, the customer focus cannot be fully delegated; you must be involved yourself.

Action Step: **Ask your managers and staff which customers they visited this month.**

Being Committed to Innovation. Externally focused leaders recognize that innovation and creativity are important concepts in effective competition. The leader is aware that the needs and expectations of customers are continually changing and that competitors continually change in an effort to capture more market share. Innovation is the only way to continually provide value to customers—by improving current services and products, developing new services and products, and increasing cost-effectiveness. To enhance innovation, set the expectation that everyone will think creatively about work and how to improve it. Reward ideas that are creative.

Action Step: **Foster innovation and creativity throughout the organization through formal and informal actions.**

Being Visible. The leader understands that he or she must be visible on the front lines. To capture employees' attention, you must build trust, describe the vision, and listen intently to problems. It is impossible to be a visible leader from your office; if you wander around the organization, you will build employees' commitment and loyalty.

Action Step: **Frequently make rounds and talk to employees throughout your organization. Ask them how things are going, rather than just saying hello.**

Being Committed to Education and Training. Leaders themselves must be lifelong learners, and they must encourage the same trait in others. Leaders recognize the importance of education and training for effective competition. Most healthcare organizations state that their most important resource is people, but there is often no visible commitment to people in the same organizations. How do you show your investment in people? Education is one way for you to show that you mean what you say. At the same time, it is a way to receive a return on your investment.

> *Action Step*: **Invest in your employees. Enhance training and development. Do a broad-based needs assessment. Ask employees what skills they need to be more effective. Design programs to meet the needs. Use management expectations to develop your programs.**

One useful approach to emphasizing the importance of education and training is to establish expectations of completed education and training programs for current and new positions.

Being Willing to Decentralize and Delegate. Because leaders recognize the need to do so, they are willing to delegate responsibility and authority. Transformation of healthcare organizations requires the talent and effort of everyone. Organizations cannot afford executives who try to retain all information and authority centrally. Effective delegation means really letting go. It is the indispensable element of empowerment, which will lead to superb performance (Peters, 1987).

Developing effective delegation skills takes time. Most managers are willing to delegate responsibility, but far fewer are willing to delegate meaningful authority to make decisions, usually because they fear the consequences of a "wrong" decision by a subordinate. Many healthcare organizations require corporate officers to approve subordinates' purchases that are as low as $1,000, yet those same subordinates manage people who cost millions of dollars per year.

What authority do departmental managers and other managers have in your organization? Limits on spending authority are usually based on uneasiness about controlling expenditures. Develop exception-reporting systems, so that if a manager is spending questionably, you can address the pattern rather than every decision. You must provide leadership to ensure that subordinates receive relevant information. Develop and share management expectations. Each manager should fully understand the attitudes and skills expected, and performance reviews should be based on those expectations. Foster a risk-taking attitude; to make change, you must have people willing to take risks. Many managers delay risky decisions, hoping that the need will go away. Today's environment will not allow "paralysis by analysis" or indecision. Champion change in your organization. Provide support for risk takers, and embrace error as a way to learn.

> *Action Step*: **Hire the best people you can and delegate effectively. Develop management expectations and provide these to all managers. Frequently ask how people are using the expectations to improve.**

Fostering Supplier Relationships. Leaders stay linked to the suppliers who provide services and products used by their organizations. Suppliers should be considered part of your team, helping you to meet your customers' requirements. Suppliers can be excellent sources of innovation to help you improve, if you and your managers work with them. Another way to improve quality is to reduce the number of suppliers. By working with fewer suppliers and articulating your needs effectively, you can develop a stronger working relationship, which will result in lower levels of service or product variation and higher levels of quality.

> *Action Step*: **Visit suppliers yourself, and request that other managers and key employees visit sup-**

pliers to discuss requirements and how they can
help. Reduce the number of suppliers.

Knowing Yourself. Leaders must constantly assess their
strengths and weaknesses and work on areas that need to be
strengthened. It is important to ask for feedback from those you
manage, to be sure that your perceptions are accurate as you
build your self-development plan. Accept the feedback, and do
not argue with people's perceptions.

Action Step: Develop the habit of asking your managers and employees what you can do to make
them more successful.

The Gap Between Management and Leadership Skills

In most healthcare organizations, there is a tremendous
gap between the skills required of managers and leaders and the
actual skills of the people in management positions. There are a
number of explanations for the gap.

Technical Training. The majority of staff members in most
healthcare organizations either are technically trained or have
had little formal education. Consider the many professionals
involved and the training they receive. Physicians, nurses, pharmacists, radiological technologists, laboratory technologists,
medical record librarians, respiratory therapists, computer pro-
grammers, accountants, biomedical engineers, and many others
have been educated as technical specialists. This is appropriate
and necessary for them to perform in those technical positions.
Others, like housekeepers, nurses' aides, orderlies, door attendants, and dietetic aides, may have had little formal education.
The problem is that neither group has been either educated
about the broader issues related to healthcare or trained in the
day-to-day skills required of managers and leaders. People are
expected to learn on the job.

Little Supplemental Management Training. Consider what happens on the job. A nurse, for example, does excellent work caring for patients and gets along well with fellow employees. That nurse is promoted to a position as head nurse and may now be responsible for a multimillion-dollar budget for staff, equipment, and supplies. Similar scenarios can apply to pharmacy managers, biomedical engineering managers, laboratory managers, housekeeping supervisors, and others. Yet few healthcare organizations provide new managers with more than a few hours of training for their new roles. It should come as no surprise that most managers in healthcare organizations are deficient in one or more of the skills of basic management, let alone the skills of a leader. Compare this situation to the one in many major business organizations, where a six-month to two-year training program is offered to new managers.

Attitudes Toward Recruitment. Many healthcare organizations take the position that they will recruit senior managers who have the required skills, yet if healthcare organizations are not willing to train managers, where will tomorrow's senior managers come from? Overall, most healthcare organizations reveal a large gap between the requirements of managers and existing skills. They lack on-the-job development programs for building management skills. We suggest using such a program for skill-building purposes (Germ and Coffey, 1983).

Developing Leadership Skills

One underlying assumption validated in the literature is that leadership skills can be learned if one is willing to invest time and energy (Kouzes and Posner, 1987). Certainly, some people are inherently more able and will become better leaders, but we believe that most healthcare managers can learn the necessary leadership skills to help their organizations compete more effectively.

Anyone can benefit from studying the skills of new management and leadership, which have been demonstrated in industry. These skills can be applied more effectively if the top executives of your organization are leading the effort. Even as a middle manager, however, one can improve the parts of the organization that one is responsible for and hope that the new behaviors and progress will be noted by people at the top.

Knowledge Expansion

For managers to become effective leaders, they must expand their knowledge in several areas. They must continually stretch themselves and reach beyond their abilities. Boring, routine jobs do not inspire growth. Build your skills and abilities by testing yourself. To make integrated decisions, leaders must have knowledge of a broad range of topics. They must be curious about life in general and must read as much as possible to keep informed.

External Awareness. Leaders must be externally focused and must develop knowledge of the environment outside the organization. You, other managers, and employees aspiring to become managers should develop awareness of external issues. One approach is to read general healthcare magazines, such as *Modern Healthcare* and *Hospitals*; general business publications, such as the *Wall Street Journal, Forbes, Time,* and *Business Week*; regional business publications, such as *Crain's Business* for different major cities; and local and regional newspapers. Participating in local and regional business organizations is another important way to develop external awareness.

> *Action Step*: **Circulate general business publications, and encourage your employees to participate in local and regional business organizations.**

A portion of the costs of membership in such organizations could be paid, as further encouragement. The objective is to learn about the national, regional, and local issues that may be affecting your organization. This broadens your knowledge as a leader and enhances your organization's competitive position.

Knowledge of Competitors. Leaders know their competitors almost as well as their own organizations. Managers should be expected to know every organization that competes with yours for every service and product in their own managerial areas. Further, managers should be familiar with the services, pricing, strengths, and weaknesses of all competitors. For example, the director of occupational therapy should know every organization in the area offering occupational therapy services, the size of the staff, the types of services offered, prices of those services, hours of service, and so on.

> *Action Step*: **Promote knowledge about competitors by distributing any information about them to managers. Ask managers about competitors who offer similar services, and periodically ask for summary reports on competitors.**

A planning or marketing department is an excellent source of this information, but departmental managers should have and understand the information, too.

Knowledge of Patient Origin and Referral Sources. Managers should also understand the origin of their patients and other customers, as well as the referral sources of those customers, if appropriate. For example, the manager of a physician's office should know the origin of all patients and who referred new patients to the practice. Referrals may be from other physicians, current patients, or community agencies.

> *Action Step*: **Discuss patient origin and referral statistics and relationships with managers and physicians, and request periodic summary reports. (A planning or marketing department can be a good source of information.)**

Market Trends and Directions. Leaders must have a keen sense of market trends and directions and their impacts on the organization. Healthcare, business, and government publications are excellent sources of such information, as well as books on future directions, like *Megatrends: Ten New Directions Transforming Our Lives* (Naisbitt, 1982) and *Can Hospitals Survive? The New Competitive Health Care Market* (Goldsmith, 1981), which provide insights into major business and healthcare directions.

> *Action Step*: **Hold at least quarterly meetings where market trends and directions and their impact on different functions of your organization are discussed.**

Leadership Skills Development

Leaders must have specific skills to accomplish the transformation of healthcare organizations. We here address some of those skills and things you can do to develop them.

Promoting a Total Quality Process. Implementing a total quality process is much more than establishing a marketing approach toward customers. An attitude of customer orientation is certainly the basis of a total quality process, but basic changes to improve processes in your organization are necessary for accomplishing other improvements. Hence, you must address both customer orientation and techniques and actions to improve processes. The best way to start is by reading and circulating books and articles on the total quality process. Books by Deming (1986), Juran (1988), Crosby (1979), and Scholtes and others (1988) are good for starters.

> *Action Step*: **Constantly reinforce the principles of continual quality improvement in your interactions with everyone. Managers and employees will learn and adapt approaches supported by their leaders.**

Reorganizing to Improve Cost-Effectiveness. Most organizations have reorganized many times during the past ten years, but some of these reorganizations have been like rearranging the chairs on the deck of the Titanic. The aims of reorganization should be to get closer to the customer, provide better quality, and become more cost-effective.

> *Action Step*: **Ask yourself and other managers about the minimum and most effective management structure to accomplish the goals. Anything more is not cost-effective.**

As described in Chapter Eight, empowerment of employees takes time, but in the end it can be both cost-effective and conducive to an enjoyable work environment. Improving leadership skill requires focusing on the processes for accomplishing that goal. The organization should then support those processes.

> *Managing Quantitative and Qualitative Information.* Although most organizations have stacks of data, managers have little skill in managing with quantitative and qualitative information. To improve their skills, you should regularly raise the following issues. First, with your managers and staff, discuss the difference between useless data and meaningful information that helps with processes. Many of the data currently available in most healthcare organizations are related to individual transactions and are of little use in managing processes. Data commonly exist in several unrelated manuals and computer systems. Hence, managers and employees have little summary information with which to make judgments about improvement.

> *Action Step*: **Ask managers and employees what information they need. Then modify information systems to collect and/or calculate that information. To avoid making decisions from one data point, produce graphs of data from several periods.**

Using graphs of data over time improves questions asked and decisions and actions taken. Developing this skill requires diligence. For example, it is far too easy to criticize a respiratory therapy director about "high" overtime last month without understanding whether that criticism is appropriate. Appropriateness can be judged only through seeing monthly overtime for the last year or more.

It is easy but inappropriate to try to collect all possible data, and it is appropriate to do special data collection for evaluating particular theories or hypotheses about improving processes. One point worth remembering is that the accuracy of data that are not used approaches zero over time. For example, if an admissions data form includes a space for the religion of the patient but no one uses that information, then clerks will take less care to get such information from patients. If you analyzed this information after a year, the results would be suspect at best.

Some of the most important decisions may be based on qualitative information and judgment. We do want quantitative information to help us make decisions, but such information is historical (or, at best, current). Leaders must predict and make decisions about the future. To develop leadership, you must allow managers to make decisions on the basis of qualitative information and judgments. You should discuss ideas, rationales, and risks carefully, to avoid irrational decisions, but you must also allow decisions to be based on qualitative information, as long as the risks are reasonable.

Promoting Success as Everyone's Role. The greater the number of people committed to success, the more likely your organization is to learn and innovate more quickly than its competitors. Promoting success as everyone's role is a valuable leadership skill. You can develop this skill in managers by raising their awareness of the contributions and abilities of people throughout the organization. You must overcome the attitude that employees just "do their jobs"; they also think and contribute.

Action Step: **Personally compliment and publicly praise employees who demonstrate creative and**

managerial responsibility. Ask managers for examples from their respective areas, as a method of calling their attention to the contributions of their employees.

A janitor or a dietetic aide, for example, may be a great Little League baseball coach, a leader in his or her church, or a writer for a social club. Raising awareness of their skills will encourage these employees to contribute to your organization. Another approach to encouraging managers to involve staff members is to ask them how many staff members have promoted the success of the organization, who they are, and what they did.

Table 6 shows an assessment form for determining leadership characteristics in yourself or others. Although this assessment has not been widely tested, it can still be useful.

Settings for Leadership Development

Leadership development can occur in a variety of settings. There are many ways to build the necessary skills.

On-the-Job Training. The job is obviously the most important setting in which to develop skills. One learns through theory and experience. A series of educational courses, experiences, and actions should be constructed to ensure development of the desired leadership skills. The same set should be used for current and new managers. Programs for current managers may have to be focused more on current activities, to retain managers' interest. Most important, behaviors must be consistent from the bottom to the top of the organization. Large organizations allow for role modeling and mentoring opportunities. Watching those who have been successful gives one an idea of what skills to expand and what behaviors may require modification.

Professional Conferences. External conferences introduce new ideas and approaches used by other organizations. Such conferences stimulate new ideas and can lead to innovation in your organization. Conferences on general business issues and

Table 6. Assessment of Leadership Characteristics.

Characteristic	Leader's Score Poor — Good
1. Has an external focus	
a. Understands the community/service area	0 1 2 3 4 5
b. Is sensitive to changes and trends in the environment	0 1 2 3 4 5
c. Demonstrates social concern and responsibility	0 1 2 3 4 5
d. Measures customers' perceptions of services and products	0 1 2 3 4 5
e. Has a network of external contacts	0 1 2 3 4 5
f. Measures progress against competitors	0 1 2 3 4 5
2. Promotes vision and values for the future	
a. Formulates a vision of the future	0 1 2 3 4 5
b. Communicates the vision and values	0 1 2 3 4 5
c. Demonstrates visible leadership toward vision and values	0 1 2 3 4 5
d. Mobilizes people to achieve the vision	0 1 2 3 4 5
3. Promotes continual quality improvement	
a. Is driven by customers' values	0 1 2 3 4 5
b. Meets with customers regularly about their requirements and process improvements	
(1) External customers	0 1 2 3 4 5
(2) Internal customers	0 1 2 3 4 5
c. Meets with suppliers regularly about requirements and process improvements	
(1) External suppliers	0 1 2 3 4 5
(2) Internal suppliers	0 1 2 3 4 5
4. Acts as a change agent	
a. Seeks innovation and new ideas	0 1 2 3 4 5
b. Sponsors and supports change	0 1 2 3 4 5
c. Creates an environment supportive of change	0 1 2 3 4 5
5. Values people	
a. Operates from an ethical framework	0 1 2 3 4 5
b. Views people as an important asset	0 1 2 3 4 5
c. Communicates well with people at all levels	0 1 2 3 4 5
d. Promotes education and training	0 1 2 3 4 5
e. Sets clear expectations	0 1 2 3 4 5
f. Motivates people positively to achieve	0 1 2 3 4 5
6. Demonstrates skills of management, especially under circumstances of uncertainty or conflict	
a. Plans	0 1 2 3 4 5
b. Organizes	0 1 2 3 4 5
c. Coordinates	0 1 2 3 4 5
d. Directs	0 1 2 3 4 5
e. Controls	0 1 2 3 4 5

Table 6. Assessment of Leadership Characteristics, Cont'd.

	Leader's Score	
Characteristic	Poor	Good
7. Decentralizes information and authority		
a. Distributes information widely	0 1 2 3 4 5	
b. Delegates responsibility and authority	0 1 2 3 4 5	
c. Empowers people throughout the organization	0 1 2 3 4 5	
8. Pursues self-development		
a. Knows self	0 1 2 3 4 5	
b. Identifies personal strengths and weaknesses	0 1 2 3 4 5	
c. Corrects or adapts to minimize weaknesses	0 1 2 3 4 5	
d. Pursues program of self-development and lifelong learning	0 1 2 3 4 5	
Number of Occurrences	_ _ _ _ _ _	
Total Score	_____	

trends outside the healthcare industry are also relevant. It is possible to develop mentoring opportunities with leaders met at conferences. Meeting someone who is a nationally recognized expert in one's field allows one to develop new skills. In your organization, you should ask people who plan to attend conferences to bring back and present ideas and products that may be useful. Then those people will attend the conference and look for such ideas.

Formal Education. On the average, people working in healthcare organizations have relatively high education levels, but few healthcare organizations actively encourage their employees and others to pursue education continually. One approach to encouraging education is to partially reimburse tuition for any courses, not just those that are related to the current job. Better-informed, broader-thinking people help contribute to innovation.

Off-the-Job Community Involvement. Community and social organizations provide an excellent setting for employees and managers to develop their management and leadership skills and stay linked to customers.

Management and Leadership Expectations

One effective method of developing management and leadership skills is to prepare a written set of management and leadership expectations. These should convey the types of attitudes and behaviors expected of managers in your organization. The expectations can also be communicated to your customers and suppliers. The process of formalizing the statements is important in gaining agreement on what your organization really expects of its managers and leaders.

Two organizations with written management expectations are the University of Michigan Hospitals (Ann Arbor) and NKC Hospitals, Inc. (Louisville, Kentucky). The management expectations for the University of Michigan Hospitals were given in Exhibit 4.

Dealing with Those Who Cannot Transform

Although it is not the desired outcome, some people cannot or will not change. Possibly one-third will assimilate the skills with minimal assistance, one-third will learn and develop the skills with help, and one-third will have difficulty developing the skills. Some simply cannot learn what is required in this new environment. Others have the ability but cannot adopt the new attitudes. Because of rapid organizational change, the abilities of some current employees may not be suitable in the transformed organization.

Do not make such decisions quickly. It may take a year or more for some managers to fully learn, understand, and use the new skills of leadership. Many middle managers will take a "wait and see" attitude, to discover whether the new expectations remain, and this is natural. They want to see whether top managers' actions reinforce their statements.

All managers should fully understand the attitudes and skills that they are expected to have. By regularly observing and interacting with managers, you can determine whether they are developing the attitudes and skills. Once you are sure that someone cannot or will not adapt, then you should arrange some alternative placement for that individual. If possible, the person should be placed in a nonmanagement role. If all else fails, it may be necessary to terminate the employee. If this is the case, an effort should be made to maintain the employee's self-esteem and income during the transition. Some organizations, including the University of Michigan Hospitals, have paid for outplacement services to help employees find alternative employment.

> *Action Step*: **Identify managers with the desired skills, those who are developing them, and those who cannot or will not develop the skills. Act accordingly.**

Two important yet difficult leadership skills are building a culture of continual improvement and promoting success as everyone's role within the organization.

Chapter Thirteen

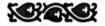

Ensuring
Organizational Excellence

The next decade offers great challenges, opportunities, and hazards. Few healthcare organizations currently have the culture or capability to make the rapid changes necessary to meet the challenges. Healthcare organizations must transform themselves, becoming more innovative and cost-effective.

Management Responsible for Transformation

Management is responsible for the success or failure of an organization. In virtually all cases, organizational failure is because of poor management. These are not comforting statements to those of us who are currently in management positions. Traditional leaders and managers tend to accept applause when things go well but blame workers or the environment when things go poorly.

Before you can transform your organization, you must transform your leaders and managers. Throughout this book, we have presented many difficult steps for improving leadership and management skills. The future of your organization depends on the knowledge, attitudes, and skills of your leaders and managers. They must be aligned before the organization can be transformed. What it really comes down to is where you as a leader focus your attention. Regularly ask your managers and staff questions about values, customers' requirements, competitors, supplier relationships, promotion of change, education and training of managers and staff, innovation, sharing information, and the business world in general. Look for responses that indicate the knowledge, attitudes, and skills you expect of leaders. Develop a document to articulate management/leadership expectations, as a way of communicating the desired and expected behaviors.

Facing the Future

It may be helpful to visualize how two organizations will face the future. First, we will look at how a traditional, non-transformed organization may face the changing environment. Second, we will look at the transformed organization, which has developed the leadership and capabilities discussed in this book. Finally, you should ask yourself where your organization is and where you would like it to be. It may be like one of the two models, or it may fall somewhere in the middle.

The traditional organization will be reactive and will wait and follow others. The managers will continue to blame employees for poor productivity and will implement increasingly punitive systems of productivity management and cost control. These actions will sow fear throughout the organization. The best employees will leave because they will find more rewarding jobs elsewhere. These losses will be most critical among nurses and the other allied health professionals who are in short supply. The remaining employees will do only the minimum to get by. The patients and medical staff will become increasingly displeased with the organization as they become aware of better quality, more cost-effectiveness, and, probably, lower-priced services elsewhere. Managers will use a series of across-the-board cost reductions in an attempt to remain profitable, but facilities, equipment, and human resources will deteriorate as depreciation funds are used to pay for operational expenses. In approximately five to fifteen years, this organization will be facing business and financial losses and will either close or be taken over by another organization.

The transformed healthcare organization will also face serious challenges. Financial constraints, rising costs, and increasing competition have made the healthcare industry risky for everyone and every organization. The difference is that the transformed organization will be proactive and will make fundamental changes in its values, culture, and leadership. It will make continual improvements in its processes, becoming customer-driven and quality-oriented. Innovation and change will be encouraged through greater employee involvement. In a word, the transformed organization will become more *responsive* to customers, market changes, reimbursement changes, employee requirements, and other factors. Leaders will communicate organizational values and will motivate others to learn and innovate faster. They will develop closer relationships with physicians, suppliers, and customers. The organization will work with others to improve its processes and achieve the best value for customers, since patients, business employers, unions, and other customers will become increasingly sensitive to the value of services and products.

Now visualize your organization, now and in five years. How prepared are you for the future? What changes do you anticipate? Are you taking appropriate actions to deal proactively with change?

Components of Transformation

We hope that you are convinced by now of the need for change. Leaders must initiate and lead the transformation. You can delegate many operating decisions and actions, but you cannot fully delegate implementation of a major organizational change. One of the major reasons why quality circles have not been effective in most organizations is that senior and middle managers delegated responsibility for implementation to lower-level managers and staff. When those people raised issues that challenged the policies or ideas of senior managers, they were not supported. It did not take long for the people involved to figure out that senior managers were not committed to change.

We have described the transformation process as involving several vital components, and we will briefly summarize some of our conclusions. The components are clearly interdependent. For example, an innovative idea may improve quality or cost-effectiveness. You may organize the components differently, but the same actions will be required.

Revitalizing Mission and Values. The organization must have clear, easily understood, and emotionally compelling vision, mission, and values. Perceived benefits must outweigh the risks and frustrations of change. Furthermore, the organization overall, and each department or entity within it, should have clearly stated goals that all employees can understand and relate to their own jobs. How can you expect managers and staff to live by the values and accomplish the goals of the organization if you do not tell them what the values and goals are or, even worse, if you do not know them yourself? Yet most healthcare organizations are doing precisely that. Publish, communicate, and ask managers and staff about the mission, values, and goals.

Establishing a Total Quality Process. As reimbursement for healthcare services becomes more standardized, healthcare providers may be competing more on quality than on price. The term *total* is used with *quality* to indicate that the approach should be applied to everything we do, not just to selected medical quality-assurance programs. The key is to identify *all* internal and external customers for *every* service, product, or process that your employees are involved with. Then talk directly with *each* customer about his or her needs, and reach an agreement on the requirements to be met. This should not be viewed as a win-lose negotiation; the idea is to reach a win-win agreement, in which both customer and supplier are satisfied. Then the goal should be to make continuing process improvements, to meet the requirements every time. Certainly errors may occur, but everyone should continually seek to make process improvements to eliminate them. A contrary concept, found in many performance plans, is that a continuing error rate (5 percent, for example) represents acceptable performance. This means that 5 percent of your customer's requirements will not be met, which violates the agreement with the customer and the principle of continual improvement.

Building a Culture of Continual Improvement. Who could argue against continual improvement? Yet few organizations actively pursue it. Most managers and organizations unwittingly try to maintain status quo. Leaders must create an environment that encourages improvement. If you regularly ask managers and staff what they have improved in the previous month, you convey a strong message: that you expect continual improvement.

Promoting Innovation and Creativity. The ability of your organization to change and continually improve is tied directly to the rate at which your organization learns and innovates. Probably one of the most important things a leader can do is to stimulate innovation. The key is to remove the personal threat of new ideas, from two perspectives. First, raising ideas should be encouraged, even if a given idea is not useful. Second, people who manage a process should not be criticized because someone else raises an idea to improve the process. Many managers resist new ideas for the latter reason. Their bosses say something like "That is a good and simple idea. Why didn't you think of it before now?" Such questions defeat innovation. A recommended approach to generating ideas and learning quickly is to have everyone pose theories for how processes can be improved. Then, simply test the ideas, to see which ones are useful.

Reorganizing the Way People Work and Interact. A key to success is changing the way work is actually accomplished. Most reorganizations of healthcare organizations simply change the management structure, without changing how work gets done. This practice is like rearranging the chairs on the deck of the *Titanic.* Reducing the management hierarchy and increasing employees' involvement are important in resolving communication problems and improving cost-effectiveness. Leaders must delegate responsibility and authority, and they must pass on information. Self-directed work groups are one effective approach, but they require substantial training and information before they can become effective. Leaders should serve as role models, mentors, and coaches, rather than as disciplinarians. They should recognize the shortage of nurses and other allied health professionals, as well as the increasing diversity of the population and the work force. Leaders of healthcare organizations should also encourage development of a multicultural environment, with education and training opportunities for everyone.

Promoting Success as Everyone's Role. Probably the most wasted resource of most healthcare organizations is the brain power of employees. The typical organization treats employees as if they left their brains at the door when they came in. Even though educational level and experience may be greater among managers, they cannot begin to generate the total number of ideas that employees can. You cannot afford to overlook the contributions of your nonmanagerial employees. The success of your organization depends on everyone's contributions. One important contribution that leaders can make is to ensure that the criteria for employees' personal success are compatible with those for the organization's success.

Improving Cost-Effectiveness. It is a simple fact that healthcare organizations must become more cost-effective. Our external environment is forcing restricted reimbursement for services and products, as well as encouraging higher expectations of quality. Cost-reduction programs being implemented by many organizations may reduce costs in the short run, but they destroy employees' morale and innovation in the long run. Cost-effectiveness should be improved through continual improvements in processes. In most cases, meaningful process improvements increase quality while they decrease costs, by eliminating steps that do not add value.

Managing with Quantitative and Qualitative Information. The need for accurate, timely, and geographically distributed information is increasing. Decision makers must have accurate information on variable and total costs of providing services or products. Bid too high, and you lose business; bid too low, and you lose money on the business you get.

Consider an increasingly common healthcare system, which consists of a hospital and a number of satellite facilities and services. Physicians and others at each facility need access to medical information from the other facilities as patients progress from the hospital to ambulatory care and possibly to home care.

Quantitative information is also needed in evaluating which of many innovative projects or theories is most useful. You need quantitative information about your competitors, as well as about your own organization. Finally, leaders must recognize that many major changes in clinical practice, technology, and social expectations will be based more on qualitative information and judgment than on historical information.

Transformation Takes Time and Courage

You should begin today, but recognize that the transformation will take years of intensive effort. The larger the organization, the longer it will take. A small group practice or a medical equipment company may be able to make a major transformation in a couple of years. At the other end of the scale, a large academic medical center may take five to ten years to make a complete transformation, because of conflicting goals. Regardless of how long transformation may take, benefits can begin immediately and will be proportional to the rate of transformation. For example, Ford Motor Company has been working on quality improvement for nine years and is still far from achieving a complete transformation, yet Ford has experienced tremendous improvements in quality, sales, and profitability.

Employees must see you and other managers demonstrating your commitment before they will significantly change their behavior. Employees will not risk change until they see evidence that managers will listen to them and support continual improvement, rather than criticizing their ideas for change.

Develop and communicate a multiyear transformation plan. Then you and other leaders must diligently implement the plan and live by its values. Certainly the plan will change, but the idea is to improve continually. Provide feedback to everyone involved in the process; everyone working on a long-term plan needs frequent feedback to avoid discouragement.

It is helpful to keep a record or diary of the methods you have used, what has succeeded, and what has failed. Such documentation stimulates the learning process, and your achievements can be communicated to others in your organization, or to other organizations.

It is up to you. Begin today! You know what you need to begin the transformation. If you are the chief executive officer, your task is clear. You can begin the actions to refocus on continual improvement. If you are not the CEO, you can still begin the change in your own area of the organization; you should not wait for the rest of the organization to change. You can have a very positive impact on your area, which may cause the rest of the organization to sit up and take notice. Widescale success, however, is unlikely without the support of the CEO. Recommend that your CEO read this book or attend a total-quality seminar with you.

Write to us, or call us, and share your successes, failures, fears, and concerns. We can all learn more rapidly as others begin the task of transforming healthcare organizations.

Resource: Action Steps of Transformation

Action steps have been listed throughout this book. These are immediate actions that you and others in your organization can take to begin implementing the principles of transformation. The action steps are listed together here, to facilitate communication about these actions among managers, staff, and others.

Chapter One: The Challenge of Organizational Excellence in Healthcare Organizations

Action Step: Become more proactive by providing regular education to the board of directors, executives, physicians, managers, employees, suppliers, and customers about the changing environment and the actions required to make improvements.

Action Step: Tell physicians, nurses, and other direct healthcare providers about financial constraints, the need to improve quality and cost-effectiveness, and the need to reduce the cost of procedures and supplies. Involve staff in planning and implementing ideas to improve quality and reduce costs.

Chapter Two: Catalysts for Change in the Healthcare Environment

Action Step: Become proactively involved in community, state, and professional organizations to seek acceptable solutions to public issues that affect healthcare organizations.

Action Step: Carefully investigate skill-mix requirements, as well as reassignment of functions performed by professional staff to nonprofessional staff. Develop strong support services, and allow the professional staff to be more productive and effective. Make sure that reassignments are cost-effective. Develop effective retention plans, to reduce turnover.

Action Step: Implement processes to continually improve quality, and develop quantitative measures of the processes and outcomes of medical care and healthcare. Without such measures, third-party payers, businesses, and patients will continue to make their decisions on the basis of price alone.

Chapter Three: Anticipating and Adapting to Changing Requirements

Action Step: Be proactive. Carefully study the environment external to your organization, to predict potential trends and changes and develop strategies to deal with them.

Action Step: Teach your management staff how to survey the external environment for signs of change that may affect healthcare and your organization. Monitor trends and new developments, and discuss them at staff meetings. Explore ways to become more proactive.

Action Step: Teach your managers what to look for, how to report information, and how to develop a plan for the future. Allow them to make valuable community contacts.

Action Step: Regularly share articles found by anyone on your staff, or designate someone to extract articles from the publications you do not regularly read, and circulate them.

Chapter Four: Revitalizing the Organization's Mission and Values

Action Step: Read your written statements of mission and goals, and answer the following questions.

1. Are the statements really clear?
2. Has every employee seen and received personal copies of these statements?
3. Do the statements address your mission and/or vision, the basic values of your organization, and the principles by which managers and staff are expected to relate to one another?
4. Do everyday activities support the mission, or is there a gap between promise and performance?

Action Step: Ask a sample of employees to read the written statements of mission and goals. Ask those employees to state in their own words what the statements mean to them. Do the employees have a clear and consistent enough understanding to use the statements on their jobs?

Action Step: With your board, physicians, customers, and managers, formally discuss the taxonomy of healthcare services, nonhealthcare ventures, and appropriate roles for your organization. Establish priorities and interrelationships with your board so that the plan will be achievable.

Action Step: Obtain formal and informal input from customers, leaders, employees, and suppliers about your mission, values, and principles. Regular input from these same groups is a key to continual improvement of quality and performance.

Action Step: Integrate the information and perceptions of others to develop clear statements of the mission, values, and principles of your organization.

Action Step: Distribute a copy of your mission and values statement to every employee, preferably on a small card that is easily carried.

Action Step: Distribute copies of the management expectations to every supervisor and manager. Review the expectations with candidates before hiring any new manager or supervisor.

Use the expectations to evaluate managers, and reward behavior in a way that is consistent with the stated expectations.

Chapter Five: Establishing a Total Quality Process

Action Step: Define *quality* as the term will be used in your organization, and communicate that definition to everyone.

Action Step: Personally promote and act in support of quality improvement, every day in every setting. In every meeting, discuss quality and process improvement.

Action Step: Begin the process of identifying customers and their requirements, throughout your organization.

Action Step: Educate managers to lead forums where employees can brainstorm about external and internal customers for the products, services, and information they provide.

Action Step: Establish one or more measurable quality-improvement goals for the most important functions of each department, and monitor progress toward quality improvement.

Action Step: For every identified quality problem, seek improvements in systems and processes first.

1. Understand and live by the organization's values and management expectations.
2. Develop missions and goals for your department(s).
3. Demonstrate commitment, sponsorship, and participation for quality improvement.
4. Identify and understand processes within your department(s) and those processes involving other departments.
5. Identify internal and external customers and suppliers for processes.
6. Determine customers' requirements.

7. Understand process capabilities.
8. Encourage ideas and theories of how to improve quality.
9. Evaluate and set priorities for opportunities.
10. Take action, if that is in your control. Use the PDCA cycle.
11. Ask for help to start an interdepartmental quality-improvement team.

Chapter Six: Building a Culture of Continual Improvement

Action Step: Understand and communicate the need and urgency for change.

Action Step: Focus attention on customers, customers' requirements, and quality.

Action Step: Develop and communicate an understanding of statistical variation.

Action Step: Provide feedback.

Action Step: Focus on process improvements.

Action Step: Focus on group or team improvements, rather than on individual accomplishments.

Action Step: Provide resources for improvement.

Action Step: Provide recognition and incentives for physicians, managers, and employees who recommend and implement changes.

Chapter Seven: Promoting Innovation and Creativity

Action Step: Teach people visualization skills.

Action Step: Complete an audit of the amount of innovative activity occurring in your organization. Ask three questions: Do your employees have degrees of freedom to do their jobs the way they think they should be done, or do they have to continually seek permission? How long does it take to implement a new idea? What rewards are there for innovators?

Action Step: Send out a call for innovative ideas, and act as a sponsor, working with intrapreneurs until projects are completed, to stimulate intrapreneurship. When success is firmly in hand, showcase results and send out another call for project proposals.

Action Step: Set up a venture-capital pool that any unit with a good idea for a new program can apply for. Structure the pool so that it becomes replenished as projects pay off. A second way you can invest in ideas is to set time aside for processing ideas and reducing potential barriers. Arrange time for employees to learn about and actually use visioning skills, to imagine their innovations and any barriers that may impede progress. Lead "what if" scenarios with your staff, to get the creative juices flowing.

Action Step: Make sure you do not fall into the trap of suppressing ideas. When people suggest ideas, help them flesh out the details. See what potential a concept has before discarding it. Show supportive behaviors when people bring ideas forward. Help them think about implementation strategies.

Action Step: Create time at staff meetings when new ideas can be presented and discussed and plans can be made for implementation.

Action Step: In your company newsletter, list all new ideas that have been implemented in the organization, along with the originators' names and any rewards.

Action Step: Review all relevant literature and information about healthcare innovation, as well as about innovations in other fields, so that new applications can be explored.

Action Step: Send copies of *The Innovators Catalog* or similar documents to your line managers for discussion at departmental meetings, to stimulate innovative thinking. Hearing about others' ideas may spark creativity. Sponsor brown-bag lunches, where people can come to share.

Action Step: Read about innovative companies, such as 3M, Hewlett-Packard, AT&T, and Wal-Mart. Learn the strategies they have used to enhance creativity and innovation.

Action Step: Nurture all creative ideas that people bring forward.

Chapter Eight: Reorganizing the Way People Work and Interact

Action Step: Begin open employee forums with the chief executive and chief operating officers, to elicit and answer employees' questions and concerns.

Action Step: Assess or evaluate your organization. Consider conducting a cultural audit to assess the institution's readiness for change.

Action Step: Develop educational brainstorming sessions, where you can outline the vision, and ask these groups to review and edit your plans for reorganizing the way work is done. Make sure you have enlisted the support of top leaders before you go public with the plans, and review the conceptual framework of the process to make sure that it is compatible with overall organizational goals.

Action Step: Develop a feasibility study. Evaluate organizational readiness for streamlining, and develop an action plan. The plan will include the strategy for implementation and an evaluation process.

Action Step: Identify key formal and informal leaders and stakeholders in your organization and educate them.

Action Step: Create a task force that can relate work reorganization to the mission, and attract volunteers to propose pilot projects in various areas of the organization.

Action Step: Provide as many opportunities for education, learning, and skill development as possible, both within your organization and in conjunction with local educational institutions. Arrange visits to corporations where teams have been functioning effectively.

Action Step: Restructure the reward system to favor team development and progress, rather than individual progress and achievement.

Action Step: Be visible and enthusiastic in supporting the team concept.

Action Step: Develop a climate where risk taking is rewarded and mistakes are viewed as opportunities for learning.

Chapter Nine: Promoting Success as Everyone's Role

Action Step: Consider restructuring the reward system for employees, with greater emphasis on group improvement and fewer evaluation categories for individuals.

Action Step: Identify the barriers that exist in your organization, and work to reduce them.

Action Step: Establish compatible organization and individual goals.

Action Step: Communicate with everyone involved.

Action Step: Recognize those who demonstrate knowledge of the values and goals.

Action Step: Solicit information on personal goals.

Action Step: Treat physicians, employees, and suppliers as partners.

Action Step: Establish two-way commitment.

Action Step: Become visibly involved in two-way communication.

Action Step: Visualize yourself in other people's situations.

Action Step: Establish trust.

Action Step: Establish an employee suggestion and/or innovation program.

Action Step: Establish a process for identifying barriers to success.

Action Step: Develop flexible systems for rewards and recognition.

Action Step: Share good and bad outcomes.

Action Step: Develop a flexible human resources system.

Chapter Ten: Improving Cost-Effectiveness

Action Step: Choose measures for each process.

Action Step: Evaluate and measure processes.

Action Step: Form a quality-improvement team.

Action Step: Make system improvements.

Action Step: Develop approved methods to accomplish each process.

Action Step: Review and revise measurement criteria.

Action Step: Develop guidelines or standards for measures.

Action Step: Develop and implement performance monitoring and reporting.

Action Step: Ask basic questions about performance.

Action Step: Manage resources to match work load and demand.

Chapter Eleven: Managing with Quantitative and Qualitative Information

Action Step: Verify that your information system can address in detail at least the following: your customers, your competitors, your suppliers, competitors of your suppliers, and alternative sources. For high-volume or high-cost items, the competition will be regional, national, or even international.

Action Step: Review your system of performance measurement, to determine whether measures exist for all key components. If not, add them.

Action Step: Decide whether and how standards will be used in your organization, and communicate that decision. If standards will be used for evaluation, extreme caution should be taken that there are agreed-upon methods to achieve the goals and the goals are acceptable to the employees.

Action Step: Verify that you are meeting the general requirements of an information system and that your system provides information both to complete service transactions and to manage the processes involved.

Action Step: Use a business-plan approach in considering data for all major decisions. A plan need not be extremely detailed for some decisions.

Action Step: Actively pursue qualitative and quantitative information that signals major changes in social expectations, clinical practice, and the economy. This information will not be available from your organization's current quantitative data.

Chapter Twelve: Rethinking Strategies for Leadership Effectiveness

Action Step: Practice visioning skills for planning purposes. Consider both personal and professional goals as opportunities.

Action Step: Discuss social responsibility of healthcare organizations at your management meetings. Give managers a chance to discuss major ethical issues.

Action Step: Demand that managers and staff present graphs of data over several periods, not data for a single period.

Action Step: Wander around the organization and ask employees what changes they have made in their units.

Action Step: Lead by example. Encourage behaviors showing that people are your most important asset. Personally serve as a coach and mentor, and encourage those who work for you to do the same.

Action Step: Encourage positive statements about your people in general, and discourage statements implying that people are easily replaceable or unimportant.

Action Step: Ask managers what specific information is being shared with employees, look for performance data posted in departments throughout the organization, and ask specific employees what information is needed.

Action Step: Visit customers yourself, and request that other managers and key employees visit their customers and discuss their requirements. Ask about your services and products, and listen to the customers' comments and concerns. Remember, the customer focus cannot be fully delegated; you must be involved yourself.

Action Step: Ask your managers and staff which customers they visited this month.

Action Step: Foster innovation and creativity throughout the organization through formal and informal actions.

Action Step: Frequently make rounds and talk to employees throughout your organization. Ask them how things are going, rather than just saying hello.

Action Step: Invest in your employees. Enhance training and development. Do a broad-based needs assessment. Ask employees what skills they need to be more effective. Design programs to meet the needs. Use management expectations to develop your programs.

Action Step: Hire the best people you can, and delegate effectively. Develop management expectations and provide these to all managers. Frequently ask how people are using the expectations to improve.

Action Step: Visit suppliers yourself, and request that other managers and key employees visit suppliers to discuss requirements and how they can help. Reduce the number of suppliers.

Action Step: Develop the habit of asking your managers and employees what you can do to make them more successful.

Action Step: Circulate general business publications, and encourage your employees to participate in local and regional business organizations.

Action Step: Promote knowledge about competitors by distributing any information about them to managers. Ask managers about competitors who offer similar services, and periodically ask for summary reports on competitors.

Action Step: Discuss patient origin and referral statistics and relationships with managers and physicians, and request periodic summary reports. (A planning or marketing department can be a good source of information.)

Action Step: Hold at least quarterly meetings where market trends and directions and their impact on different functions of your organization are discussed.

Action Step: Constantly reinforce the principles of continual quality improvement in your interactions with everyone. Managers and employees will learn and adopt approaches supported by their leaders.

Action Step: Ask yourself and other managers about the minimum and most effective management structure to accomplish the goals. Anything more is not cost-effective.

Action Step: Ask managers and employees what information they need. Then modify information systems to collect and/or calculate that information. To avoid making decisions from one data point, produce graphs of data from several periods.

Action Step: Personally compliment and publicly praise employees who demonstrate creative and managerial responsibility. Ask managers for examples from their respective areas, as a method of calling their attention to the contributions of their employees.

Action Step: Identify managers with the desired skills, those who are developing them, and those who cannot or will not develop the skills. Act accordingly.

References

Ajemian, R. "Master of the Games." *Time*, Jan. 7, 1985, pp. 32–39.

Ansberry, C. "Dumping the Poor: Despite Federal Law, Hospitals Still Reject Sick Who Can't Pay." *Wall Street Journal*, Nov. 29, 1988, pp. 1, A11.

Bass, B. M. *Leadership and Performance Beyond Expectations.* New York: Free Press, 1985.

Beckham, J. D. "Winners: Strategies of Ten of America's Most Successful Hospitals." *Healthcare Forum Journal*, Nov./Dec. 1989, pp. 17–23.

Bell, C. W. "Winners Need Stable Lineups." Editorial. *Modern Healthcare*, Dec. 2, 1988, p. 19.

Bennis, W., and Nanus, B. *Leaders: The Strategies for Taking Charge.* New York: Harper & Row, 1985.

Bice, M. O. "The Transformation of Lutheran Health Systems." In R. H. Kilmann, T. J. Covin, and Associates, *Corporate Transformation: Revitalizing Organizations for a Competitive World.* San Francisco: Jossey-Bass, 1987.

Bisesi, M. "SMR Forum: Strategies for Successful Leadership in Changing Times." *Sloan Management Review*, 1983, *25* (1), 61–64.

Block, P. *The Empowered Manager: Positive Political Skills at Work.* San Francisco: Jossey-Bass, 1987.

Bradford, D. L., and Cohen, A. R. *Managing for Excellence: The Guide for High Performance in Contemporary Organizations.* New York: Wiley, 1984.

Burns, J. M. *Leadership.* New York: Harper & Row, 1978.

Canadian Department of National Health and Welfare. *A Taxonomy of the Canadian Health Care System.* Ottawa, Ontario,

272

Canada: Health Facilities Design, Health Resources Director-
ate, Health Services and Promotion Branch, Department of
National Health and Welfare, 1979.

Carroll, L. *Alice's Adventures in Wonderland and Through the Looking-
Glass.* London: Macmillan, 1921. Reprinted by University
Microfilms, Inc., Ann Arbor, MI, p. 89.

Coffey, R. J., Gialanella, J., and Gilbert, N. E. "Decision Support
Systems: A New Role for Management Engineers." *Healthcare
Information Management,* 1989, *3* (2), 4–7.

Coile, R. C., Jr. "Macrotrends for 1990." *Osteopathic Hospital Leadership,* Dec. 1986a, pp. 8–11.

Coile, R. C., Jr. *The New Hospital: Future Strategies for a Changing
Industry.* Rockville, Md.: Aspen Systems Publishers, 1986b.

Conger, J. A., Kanungo, R. N., and Associates. *Charismatic Leadership: The Elusive Factor in Organizational Effectiveness.* San
Francisco: Jossey-Bass, 1988.

Crosby, P. B. *Quality Is Free: The Art of Making Quality Certain.* New
York: McGraw-Hill, 1979.

D'Aquila, R. "Focus on Innovation: Profiles in Creativity."
Healthcare Forum Journal, November/December 1988, p. 12.

deBono, E. *Lateral Thinking: Creativity Step by Step.* New York:
Harper & Row, 1970.

Deming, W. E. *Out of the Crisis.* Cambridge: Center for Advanced
Engineering Study, Massachusetts Institute of Technology,
1986.

Dine, D. D. "Project Involves Businesses to Make Research Mar-
ketable." *Modern Healthcare,* Feb. 24, 1989, p. 64.

Donabedian, A. *Explorations in Quality Assessment and Monitoring.*
Vol. I: *The Definition of Quality and Approaches to Its Assessment.*
Ann Arbor, Mich.: Health Administration Press, 1980.

Drucker, P. *Innovation and Entrepreneurship: Practice and Principles.*
New York: Harper & Row, 1985.

Drucker, P. "The Coming of the New Organization." *Harvard
Business Review,* Jan. 1988, pp. 45–53.

Feigenbaum, A. V. "ROI: How Long Before Quality Improvement
Pays Off?" *Quality Progress,* February 1987, pp. 32–35.

Florida Power and Light. *Team Leader Training Course Participant
Workbook.* (2nd ed.) Miami: Florida Power and Light, 1990.

273

Gallivan, M. "Inflationary Pressures Run Mergers Full." *Hospitals*, Feb. 5, 1988, p. 40.

Garvin, D. A. *Managing Quality: The Strategic and Competitive Edge.* New York: Free Press, 1988.

Germ, J. A., and Coffey, R. J. *Applied Management Programs for Managers.* Naperville, Ill.: JNS Associates, 1983.

Ginzberg, E. "Eight Facts of Life Shaping Health Care." *Hospitals*, Aug. 20, 1987, p. 80.

Gitlow, H. S., and Gitlow, S. J. *The Deming Guide to Quality and Competitive Position.* Englewood Cliffs, N.J.: Prentice-Hall, 1987.

GOAL/QPC. *Memory Jogger: A Pocket Guide of Tools for Continuous Improvement.* Methuen, Mass.: GOAL/QPC, 1988.

Goldsmith, J. G. *Can Hospitals Survive? The New Competitive Health Care Market.* Homewood, Ill.: Dow Jones–Irwin, 1981.

Greene, J. "Change Management: Hospitals Are Learning to Make the Most of Change." *Modern Healthcare*, Nov. 25, 1988, pp. 20–31.

Healthcare Forum. *Innovators Catalog.* San Francisco: Healthcare Forum, 1988.

Hickman, C. R., and Silva, M. A. *Creating Excellence: Managing Corporate Culture, Strategy, and Change.* Ontario, N.Y.: New American Library, 1984.

Hoerr, J., Pollack, M., and Whiteside, D. E. "Management Discovers the Human Side of Automation." *Business Week*, Sept. 29, 1986, pp. 70–74.

Hospital Corporation of America. *Hospitalwide Quality Improvement Process, Strategy for Improvement, FOCUS-PDCA.* Nashville, Tenn.: Hospital Corporation of America, 1989.

Imai, M. *Kaizen—The Key to Japan's Competitive Success.* New York: Random House, 1986.

Ishikawa, K. *What Is Total Quality Control? The Japanese Way.* Englewood Cliffs, N.J.: Prentice-Hall, 1985.

Johnston, W. B., and Packer, A. E. *Workforce 2000: Work and Workers for the 21st Century.* Washington, D.C.: U.S. Department of Labor, 1987.

Juran, J. M. *Juran on Quality Leadership: How to Go from Here to There.* Wilton, Conn.: Juran Institute, 1987.

Juran, J. M. *Juran on Planning for Quality*. New York: Free Press, 1988.

Kaiser, L. R. "Futurism in Health Care." *Hospital Forum*, 1980, *23* (7), 26–28.

Kaiser, L. R. "Futurism, Part II — Application." *Hospital Forum*, 1981a, *24* (2), 20–23.

Kaiser, L. R. "Futurism, Part II — Application (Continued)." *Hospital Forum*, 1981b, *24* (3), 61–68.

Kanter, R. M. *The Change Masters*. New York: Simon & Schuster, 1983.

King, B. *Better Designs in Half the Time: Implementing QFD Quality Function Deployment in America*. (3rd ed.) Methuen, Mass.: GOAL/QPC, 1989.

Kirby, T. *The Can-Do Manager: How to Get Your Employees to Take Risks, Take Action, and Get Things Done*. New York: AMACOM, 1989.

Kouzes, J. M., and Posner, B. Z. *The Leadership Challenge: How to Get Extraordinary Things Done in Organizations*. San Francisco: Jossey-Bass, 1987.

Labich, K. "Making Over Middle Managers." *Fortune*, May 8, 1989, pp. 58–64.

Mackenzie, R. A. "The Management Process in 3-D." *Harvard Business Review*, Nov./Dec. 1969, pp. 80–87.

McManis, G. L. "Transitioning from Retail to Wholesale Marketing." *Health Care Executive*, July/Aug. 1988, p. 31.

Maryland Hospital Association. *Report to Members of the Board of Trustees*. Luterville, Md.: Maryland Hospital Association, 1987.

Maynard, H. B. (ed.). *Industrial Engineering Handbook*. (3rd ed.) New York: McGraw-Hill, 1971.

Morooka, K. Presentation to GOAL/QPC, Boston, Dec. 5, 1989.

Naisbitt, J. *Megatrends: Ten New Directions Transforming Our Lives*. New York: Warner Books, 1982.

Naisbitt, J., and Aburdene, P. *Reinventing the Corporation*. New York: Warner Books, 1985.

O.D. Resources, Inc. *Change Resistance Scale*. Atlanta, Ga.: O.D. Resources, Inc., 1988.

Perot, H. R. "Perot's Manifesto." *Detroit News*, Jan. 29, 1988, pp. 1A, 4A.

Peters, T. *Thriving on Chaos: Handbook for a Management Revolution.* New York: Harper & Row, 1987.

Peters, T., and Austin, N. *A Passion for Excellence: The Leadership Difference.* New York: Warner Books, 1985.

Peters, T. J., and Waterman, R. H., Jr. *In Search of Excellence.* New York: Harper & Row, 1982.

Pinchot, G., III. *Intrapreneuring.* New York: Harper & Row, 1985.

Price, C. "Innovators and Entrepreneurs: 1989." *Hospitals*, May 20, 1989, pp. 40–54.

Raske, K. E., and Eisenman, D. "Hospitals Under the Regulatory Knife: Directions in Medical Malpractice." *New York State Journal of Medicine*, July 1986, pp. 356–360.

Rothman, E. D. Lectures on tools and techniques for quality improvement, presented at University of Michigan Hospitals, Ann Arbor, 1989.

Sabatino, F. "What Is Leadership? What's Impeding It?" *Hospitals*, May 20, 1987, pp. 52–56.

Schick, F. L. (ed.). *Statistical Handbook on Aging Americans.* Phoenix, Ariz.: Oryx Press, 1986.

Scholtes, P. R., and others. *The Team Handbook.* Madison, Wis.: Joiner Associates, 1988.

Smalley, H. E. *Hospital Management Engineering: A Guide to the Improvement of Hospital Management Systems.* Englewood Cliffs, N.J.: Prentice-Hall, 1982.

Solovy, A. "As Margins Fall, Executives Forge Survival Tools." *Hospitals*, Mar. 20, 1988a, pp. 48–52.

Solovy, A. "Cutting Out the Middlemen." *Hospitals*, November 20, 1988b, pp. 52–57.

Spechler, J. W. *When America Does It Right: Case Studies in Service Quality.* Norcross, Ga.: Industrial Engineering and Management Press, 1988.

Stansbury, J. A. Presentation on total-quality management at NKC, Inc., Louisville, Ky., Jan. 5, 1989.

Starr, P. *The Social Transformation of American Medicine.* New York: Basic Books, 1982.

Steiber, S. R. "How Consumers Perceive Health Care Quality." *Hospitals*, Apr. 5, 1988, p. 84.

Steinberg, E. P. "The Impact of Regulation and Payment Innovations on Acquisition of New Imaging Technologies." *Radiologic Clinics of North America*, 1985, *23* (3), 381–389.

Taylor, J. C., and Asodorian, R. A. "The Implementation of Excellence: STS Management." *Industrial Management*, July-Aug. 1985, pp. 5–15.

Thorsrud, E. "Policy Making as a Learning Process." In A. B. Cherns, R. Sinclair, and W. J. Jenkins (eds.), *Social Science and Government: Politics and Problems.* London: Tavistock, 1972.

Thurber, J. *The 13 Clocks.* New York: Simon & Schuster, 1950.

Tichy, N. M., and Devanna, M. A. *The Transformational Leader.* New York: Wiley, 1986a.

Tichy, N. M., and Devanna, M. A. "The Transformational Leader." *Training & Development Journal*, July 1986b, pp. 27–32.

Tichy, N., and Nisberg, J. N. "When Does Restructuring Work? Organizational Innovations at Volvo and G.M." *Organizational Dynamics.* 1976, *5* (1), 63–70.

Toffler, A. *Future Shock.* New York: Random House, 1970.

Tomasko, R. M. *Downsizing: Reshaping the Corporation for the Future.* New York: American Management Association, 1987.

Touche Ross & Company. "Survey of Hospital Executives." *Health Week*, July 5, 1988, p. 1.

Townsend, P. *Further Up the Organization.* New York: Knopf, 1984.

Trist, E., and Bamforth, K. W. *Some Social and Psychological Consequences of the Long Wall Method of Goal Getting in Human Relations.* London: Tavistock, 1951.

U.S. Department of Labor. *Opportunity 2000: Creative Affirmative Action Strategies for a Changing Work Force.* Washington, D.C.: U.S. Department of Labor, 1988.

Vraciu, R. A. "Hospital Strategies for the Eighties: A Mid-Decade Look." *Health Care Management Review*, 1985, *10* (4), 9–19.

Walton, M. *The Deming Management Method.* New York: Putnam, 1986.

Wilensky, G. R. "Cost Containment Affects Access to New Technology." *Hospitals*, Apr. 5, 1988, p. 16.

Zaleznek, A. "Managers and Leaders: Are They Different?" *Harvard Business Review*, May/June 1977, pp. 67–78.

Zinn, T. K., and DiGiulio, L. W. "Actualizing System Benefits: Part I." *Computers in Healthcare*, Mar. 1988, p. 32.

Index